"*Good Morning Intentions* is a spiritual eli
and spirit. Britt and Tara have created a p
cultivate a sacred space for your soul to be nurtured, supported, and
loved. Each ritual presents a unique offering that will transform and
enrich your life."
    —AUSTYN WELLS, GC-C, spiritual medium,
    and award-winning author of *Soul Conversations*

"As a longtime devotee of the morning ritual practice, I was inspired
to expand my personal rituals using Britt and Tara's combinations
of mantras, mudras, yoga, meditations, and affirmations. As I used
them, I felt more at peace and centered than ever, with all the cobwebs
cleared out. *Good Morning Intentions* is a high-vibration treasure."
    —LISA CAMPION, Reiki master teacher,
    and author of *The Art of Psychic Reiki*

"What better way to start your day on a positive note than a series of
morning rituals that help you focus on growth and self-care? In *Good
Morning Intentions*, Britt Deanda and Tara Schulenberg serve as
insightful guides to caring for body, mind, and spirit with meaningful
rituals to energize your intentions. Choose one ritual or try them all.
You'll be better for having done so."
    —KAREN FRAZIER, intuitive energy healer,
    Reiki master, and author of *The Crystal Alchemist*

"Britt and Tara came into my life at the most serendipitous time, and
introduced the magic of Kundalini yoga into my life. They are two
of the brightest, most shining spirits that I know, and everything
they do is so full of love, high vibrations, and pure intention. This
book is no exception. There is magic woven into every word,
ritual, meditation, and story shared in this beautiful book. You are
guaranteed to feel more centered and awakened after reading—there
is no doubt in my mind!"
    —JORDAN YOUNGER, creator of The Balanced Blonde, host of
    the top-rated *Soul On Fire* podcast, author, and spiritual teacher

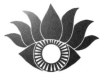

GOOD MORNING INTENTIONS

Sacred Rituals to Raise Your Vibration, Find Your Bliss & Stay Energized All Day

BRITT DEANDA

TARA SCHULENBERG

NEW HARBINGER PUBLICATIONS, INC.

Publisher's Note

This publication is designed to provide accurate and authoritative information in regard to the subject matter covered. It is sold with the understanding that the publisher is not engaged in rendering psychological, financial, legal, or other professional services. If expert assistance or counseling is needed, the services of a competent professional should besought.

Medical Disclaimer: *The ideas, yogic postures, procedures, and suggestions in this book are not intended as a substitute for professional medical advice from a trained health professional. Before you begin any exercise or health program and before adopting the suggestions in this book, please always consult your physician, as well as about any condition that may require diagnosis or medical attention. The benefits attributed to the practice of Kundalini yoga and meditation stem from centuries-old yogic tradition. Results will vary with individuals. Neither the author or the publisher shall be liable or responsible for any loss, injury, or damage allegedly arising from any information or suggestion in this book.*

Printed in China

Distributed in Canada by Raincoast Books

Cover design by Sara Christian. Acquired by Elizabeth Hollis Hansen. Edited by Gretel Hakanson. Text design by Amy Shoup. All Rights Reserved. Cover photo by Brooke Cagle on Unsplash. Illustrations by Miray Yalcinkaya. Interior photos by Alina Karpenko on Unsplash (p. vi), Ashley Streff (p. 2), Grant Durr on Unsplash (p. 12), Liam Pozz on Unsplash (p. 38), Erol Ahmed on Unsplash (p. 72), Ameenfahmy on Unsplash (p. 98), Carolyn V on Unsplash (p. 126), Krystal Ng on Unsplash (p. 154), and Sacha Styles on Unsplash (p. 190).

Library of Congress Cataloging-in-Publication Data

TK

22   21   20

10 9 8 7 6 5 4 3 2 1   First Printing

We are the people who put inner freedom first.

Who love beyond all else.

Who aim to uplift the people in front of us, beside us, and behind us.

Who wake up and expect miracles.

Who see the world as our family.

Who live intuitively connected to ourselves and Mother Earth.

We are cocreators of our lives and the planet.

We are here to break the rules that bind people to lower levels of consciousness.

To help humanity rise.

We don't just live for ourselves.

We work for the light.

Contents

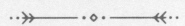

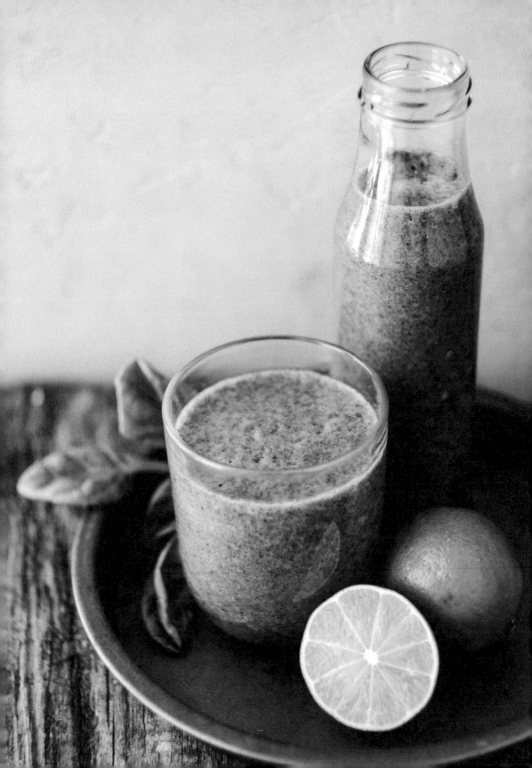

Welcome to an Elevated Start, Every Day

We have a question for you: Are you in the driver's seat of your own life, making each day a masterpiece and chasing after your wildest dreams? Or are you sitting in the passenger seat, just watching the scenery pass you by?

If you're riding shotgun, you're not alone. In fact, we were both there not that long ago. It's so easy to get caught up in the chaos of modern life—endless work emails, negative news headlines, dating and relationship struggles, money worries, and the pull between putting organic veggies on your plate and meeting up with friends over mimosas at brunch. It can feel like you're playing a daily game of whack-a-mole, reacting to the events of life versus cocreating them.

You may expend so much energy on this game that you go to extreme measures to cheer yourself up. (We certainly used to.) Whether it's drugs, alcohol, codependent relationships, reality TV, or online shopping binges, distractions like these cause us to completely miss the blessings of the moment and keep us from actually enjoying and realizing what a freaking gift it is to wake up and be alive!

Sound familiar? Well, no matter where you are on your path, we're here to show you what's possible when you become a conscious creator of your own life in a bigger way, taking back control of the steering wheel and setting your GPS toward your destiny. To get back in the driver's seat, you must have the energy, determination, courage, confidence, self-authority, and self-love to sustain you.

In our experience, the fastest and most effective way to do this is by adopting a consistent morning ritual—rising with the sun and doing a daily spiritual practice that lights you up, keeps your energetic vibration on point, and keeps your intuition clear, no matter what life throws at you. When you start your day by connecting deeply to yourself, your inner compass can direct you toward your highest path. You have the strength and energy to take care of yourself and others. You become a warrior for happiness and love, following the wild desires in the back of your mind and creating the internal source of positive energy that helps you take aligned action toward your goals.

Morning rituals guide you to tap into the deeper experience available beyond the five senses and the physical human world. We are all spiritual beings having a human experience, but sometimes we get that mixed up. So we are here to remind you of your deep connection to your soul—get ready to become BFFs with your spirit!

Meet Your Guides, Britt + Tara

We are so honored to connect and share these rituals with you, and we can't wait to get to know each other through this work. We know *all* about the benefits of good morning intentions because we experience them every day—and we are excited for you to experience them as well!

We both started waking up to the power of a daily spiritual practice when we started shifting our lifestyle and eventually became certified Kundalini yoga instructors. In the years since, we've crafted super-powerful morning ritual formulas of our own—including practices from Kundalini yoga and meditation, manifestation techniques, self-care, and plant-based nutrition. They were so life-changing for us that we now have to share them with the world.

We credit this game-changing practice with empowering us to leave our corporate jobs, release addictions and other unhealthy patterns, and step into our power as spiritual leaders and founders of Elevate the Globe, our spiritual lifestyle brand with the mission to elevate all of humanity, one person at a time, through daily spiritual practices.

Thanks to the clarity and energy we get from our morning rituals, we've achieved our wildest dreams: We work in our yoga pants, speaking, writing, and teaching Kundalini yoga and other high-vibrational concepts to thousands of people; we share our truth and interview amazing humans on our podcast, *The Elevator*; we host retreats in Bali and travel the world to teach; we've created several online courses and a membership community that inspire people to upgrade their health, relationships, and abundance in unbelievable ways; and now we get to share this book with you! Most of all, we have found incredible amounts of happiness, joy, and peace in just being alive, and that is what we want you to experience because, as humans, we all deserve happiness. If you want to read more about where we came from and how we got here, go to http://www.newharbinger.com/45724 for our personal stories.

Our intention with this book is to give you twenty-one morning rituals that will enhance every area of your life. The theme and elements of each ritual—including the Kundalini yoga and meditation—were curated by us with guidance from what we call Source. (You may call it the Divine, God, the Universe, or some other wonderful name.) Many of the themes within this book are common areas of interest across our Elevate the Globe community, and the rituals often arrived to us during our own morning rituals as visions or ideas from our spirit guides and Source! Kundalini yoga is believed to have been around and practiced for thousands of years, and bringing it to a broader audience in the form of fun morning rituals is the most beautiful exchange we can imagine at this time in our lives.

Why the Morning in "Morning Ritual"?

Okay, we know what you're thinking—you barely have enough time to get out the door in the morning as it is, right? Or maybe you have some sort of ritual, but it's not consistent or uber effective. Don't stress; it's not just you. We know it can be really hard to think about squeezing *another* task into your a.m. hours, but we promise that if you create the space and time to do so, it will be well worth the reward!

There are a few reasons why we recommend doing your spiritual practice first thing in the morning. In the Kundalini yoga tradition, the two and a half hours before sunrise are called the "ambrosial hours," or *amrit vela*. This is when the electromagnetic energy of the Earth is said to optimally support meditation. The rising sun's rays are infrared and attuned to the longer "theta" waves of your dreamtime brain, which is the same state of the brain in deep meditation. What that means is the waves of sunlight align with the waves of our meditation, which aligns us with heightened levels of subconscious clearing and increased clarity and intuition. Translation: it's a time for meditation on natural sunny steroids.

In the ancient Indian medical tradition of Ayurveda, the early morning hours—from 2:00 to 6:00 a.m.—are when the mental energies of purity and lightness are most present. We like to call it "magic energy" because it helps us drop into a contemplative state deeper and faster. We're all about that efficiency!

If you need science to convince you to give up the snooze button, there's plenty of research showing the benefits of waking up early. A 2008 study in the *Journal of General Psychology* found that early risers procrastinate less than those who stay up late.[1] Harvard University researchers have discovered that those who wake up early are better at anticipating and minimizing the problems they face during the day.[2] And it's not just about what time you set your alarm for, but what you do with that extra time. In Tim Ferris's book *Tools of Titans*, more than 80 percent of the world-class performers interviewed said they practice some type of mindfulness every morning.[3]

Another benefit to starting a predawn morning practice? That's when the world is quietest. Most people are still sleeping, and your mind hasn't been inundated with a hundred work emails, kids that need you, or pets that need to be walked. It's a time when you can align with *you first*—with your energetic frequency, who you are and who you want to be, your *Sat Naam* (aka your true self)—before anything else can distract you.

When you focus your first few hours on connecting to yourself instead of your phone (and all of the other distractions present in this Aquarian Age), you're able to consciously map out the highest path for your day. We think of it like having a team meeting with the universe and all of our angels and guides. Those moments of being present create a point of connection with your highest truth, elevating you into the flow of higher energy that will carry you throughout your day.

Oh, and one more thing: it really is important to commit to your morning ritual and make it an everyday thing. It takes practice to develop consistency and mastery over yourself. The idea of commitment freaks a lot of people out, but it actually gives your subconscious mind security and love. When your mind and body start to trust you're taking care of them, you're able to enter into a state of calm surrender where you're riding the cocreation train with the universe to high places!

To get the results you want, you must allow the energy of the morning ritual to build and become a habit. That way, you can get off the bull ride that keeps bucking you into the mud and progressively move up into a higher emotional vibration.

Kundalini Yoga 101

If you are new to meditating or Kundalini yoga, just know that we make it super easy to pick up, so don't worry! Here are a few tips and terms to get you started.

Easy Pose. Typically, in Kundalini meditation and some yoga postures, we sit in Easy Pose—a simple cross-legged position on the floor. (You'll read this phrase a lot in the rituals that follow.) In Easy Pose, it's important to lengthen your spine and slightly tuck your chin so your spine is straight in the neck area. Your hands can rest on your knees, palms facing up. If you feel like your legs are falling asleep, you can periodically switch the leg that's on top or shake out both legs in front of you. Like anything, the more you do it, the more flexible you will get, and the easier it will be.

If sitting in a cross-legged position is not an option for you, you can always sit up against a wall, on a meditation cushion that raises your hips, or in a chair with your feet flat on the ground. Feel free to use these modifications, as it is most important to be comfortable and feel good.

Tuning in. At the beginning of every Kundalini class, we tune in with the "Adi Mantra" chant, which is pronounced "Ong Namo Guroo Dayv Namo." The word "Ong" calls on the creative energy within you, "Namo" means to bow to that creative energy, "Guroo" means teacher, one who brings us from darkness into light, and "Dayv" means subtle or divine. Together, "Guroo Dayv Namo" calls on the divine teacher and creative force within to guide us. This is a very powerful chant that connects you to your inner wisdom and unlocks your own beautiful energy so it can shine through you! You can find a version of this sound current on the Spotify playlist that accompanies this book called "Ong Namo (Tune In)" by Serena Savitri Kaur from the album *Dil Se* (*From the Heart*).

Timing. Kundalini yoga meditations all have very specific recommended time limits, and it's important to stick to them. But this isn't hard! All you need to do is set the timer on your computer or phone for the time specified in the ritual. Then, when it goes off, complete any of the instructions for ending the practice. (Usually, this involves taking a few deep breaths, but it varies based on the meditation.)

Dizziness and tingles. If you ever feel dizzy during a meditation, check your posture—you may just need to make sure your chin is tucked down and back so your neck is completely straight, which allows the energy you're generating to flow freely up and down your spine. Also, feel free to take a break! We find it helpful to place our hands on the floor for grounding. Take as long as you need, and then come back into the meditation. Sometimes you may also feel a buzzy, tingling energy in other parts of your body. This sometimes happens with Kundalini yoga—you are just feeling your energy vibrating, and sometimes it is a physical sign that your energy is moving, releasing, or recalibrating. Always use your intuition on how often you need to take breaks, but know that some sensations are part of the process.

Head coverings. In the Kundalini tradition, you will often see people wearing head coverings like turbans and scarves. The reason is that it helps contain the energy that's generated by the practice, which may sometimes give people a headache or an overly activated crown chakra. We don't always wear head coverings, but we often do—especially when we are doing longer meditations or practices. If you ever feel a lot of energy at the top of your head or feel a headache coming on, a head covering (even a beanie or sunhat) is highly suggested.

White clothing. We love to wear white when practicing because it expands the aura, helps deflect negativity, and is known to lift depression and elevate mood. White clothing also helps increase your awareness of your surroundings for multiple reasons—for one, you're more careful not to spill things on yourself!

The forty-day rule. Lastly, we recommend practicing any given ritual for a minimum of forty days. At the forty-day point, Kundalini yoga wisdom states that you will break any negative habits that block you from expansion. For deeper benefits, you can always go on and do these practices for 90, 120, or 1,000 days and beyond if you feel called to!

The Anatomy of the Morning Rituals

Throughout all the rituals in this book, you will find there is a general structure in common. We designed it this way because the Elevate the Globe lifestyle is not just single-faceted—it's a holistic approach. Before you dive into your first ritual, take a look at the different elements included and the "why" behind them.

Setting up your meditation space with a yoga mat or cushion. Having a designated sacred space to do your practice helps you turn it into a ritual you'll look forward to—and you won't have to decide where you are going to do your practice when you wake up! Feel free to have flowers, candles, a little altar, or any inspiring photos or images that you'd like to see every day. This is a great place to keep any crystals or oils you are using with your ritual.

A suggested crystal and essential oil to work with. We love working with crystals and oils to enhance the energy and mind-set work we are doing! They are powerful tools that assist us in positively interacting with our body's energy field and chakras, supercharging the ritual's benefits even more! So we've included our recommendations.

Listen to mantras so you can chant along. We created a Spotify playlist to accompany this book so you can listen to the sublime sounds of some amazing musicians as you chant each mantra. Once you have the Spotify app, search for "Good Morning Intentions," *et voila!* A song for your ritual.

Breathwork. We open up many of the rituals with breathwork, otherwise known as *pranayama,* which brings more oxygen to all of our cells and helps clear the mind and get us into those theta brain waves, stat!

Warm-up. Next, we warm up with Kundalini postures and movements designed to stretch and open the body, energize the chakra energy centers, and wake up the cells. These are part of the Kundalini energy work technology and give us specific results related to each ritual while prepping us for the meditation.

Meditation. In Kundalini yoga, there are thousands of meditations, or *kriyas*, that work with different parts of our mind, body, and energy field to shift energy and create transformation. We chose meditations for each ritual that are designed to target what you are working on energetically. If you are new to meditation, these can feel a little weird and wacky, but they are very potent and effective and work fast to create the change you want! We are so honored to share these sacred meditations with you that have changed our lives and the lives of so many others.

Visualization and journaling. This mind-set work is the perfect complement to the energy work because we have found we need both. Mind-set work helps keep you on track throughout the day and gets your mind behind your "why" and what you want. It's our secret combination that works wonders!

Self-care. With all of this amazing energy and mind-set work, we also use ancient yogic self-care practices to accompany and uplevel our practices. If you need to do this part at another time throughout the day, feel free, but we highly recommend taking advantage of these simple ways to up your self-care game that are specific to each ritual.

Nourishment through high-vibrational food. Lastly, we want our post-ritual nutrition to support all of the amazing work we just did. What we eat has a huge effect on how we feel, so we curated foods and drinks that perfectly align and assist the rituals. Food is another tool that can help you achieve the transformation and goals you are going for, and these recipes are super easy to make, energizing, and delicious. We suggest using organic ingredients where possible. Enjoy!

TIPS FOR YOUR PRACTICE

- To begin, we suggest choosing the ritual that you are most called to—the one that you feel is the highest priority for you to work with first—and commit to that for forty days.

- Have no clue where to start? You can use these pages like a tarot deck—breathe deep, flip to a page, and then see if that ritual resonates with you.

- After finishing your first forty days of any ritual, you can continue with it longer if you feel called to or choose another one to work with!

- If you're short on time one day and can't complete the whole ritual in one sitting, we suggest at the very least tuning in and practicing the meditation, and if you have a little more time, add the warm-ups and the breathwork, and you can practice the other components of the ritual throughout the day or before bed.

- You can always connect to other people in the community through the Elevate the Globe Facebook group and on Instagram, as we all benefit from receiving and giving support.

Adopt a Morning Ritual, Light Up Your Life

Thousands of Elevate the Globe (ETG) community members are already riding the morning-ritual train. We hear stories all the time about people who've adopted a morning ritual to help manage their anxiety, PTSD, or post-partum depression; to help navigate addictions like smoking, drinking, and codependency; to get clear on what they wanted in a soul mate or twin-flame relationship; to attract business opportunities with the help of divine guidance from the universe; and to feel vibrant in everything they do. Whatever your intention is for doing these rituals, know that most people experience positive changes from them.

Through the journey of writing this book, we've gone deeper with our own morning rituals than ever before. Our new normal is waking up at 4:00 a.m. to meditate for two hours, which we never would have imagined possible a few years ago. Of course, we're not expecting you to do the same thing right away. Even three minutes of meditation in the morning can be really powerful! Just know that there will always be new layers to uncover—and the key is to start with where you are and grow from there.

You may have heard the saying, "The definition of insanity is doing the same thing over and over again, but expecting different results." So, are you ready to commit to this path and create the badass life you've been envisioning? It's time for new practices that catapult you into a more empowered state of being. It's time for us as a collective to engage in daily habits that support a way of living that is above the drama, is high in consciousness, and gives us that oomph of energy that makes us think, *OMG, pinch me, I can't believe this is my life*. (And we're going to have the best time doing it—get ready...go!)

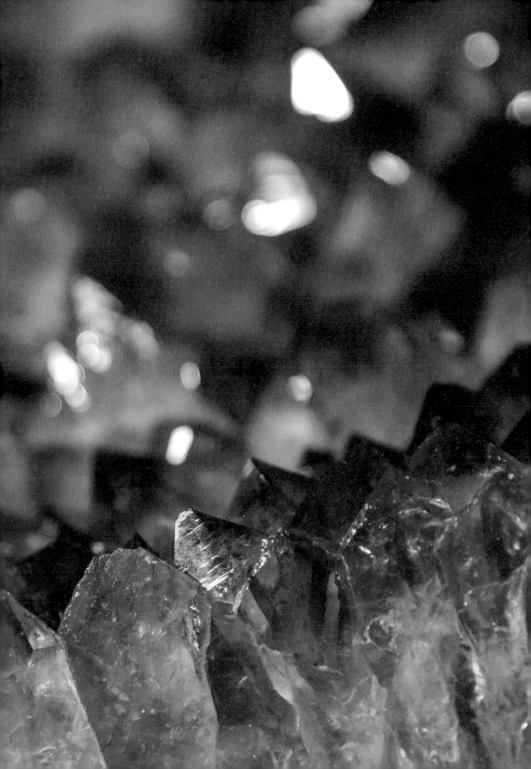

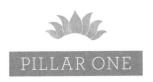

Stress Management

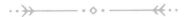

You may notice that when you're under a lot of stress, your daily routines start to feel like the beginning (or end) of the life you never wanted. Those bad habits you thought you were done with—skipping the gym, not eating healthy, letting the dishes pile up in the sink? Before you realize it, they've crept back in, and all of a sudden you're dealing with them all over again. Super frustrating, right?

Well, falling back into old patterns is just one side effect of stress—our own worst enemy. It messes with our willpower, causes hormonal changes in our bodies, and weakens our energetic fields, making it easier for us to default to bad habits. The word "stress" by definition means pressure or tension exerted on a material object—in this case, your body, your mind, and your psyche. Imagine your entire being thrown in a pressure cooker. What happens? It creates so much pressure on the body and mind that it throws you into survival mode. Anything that takes more of your energy to maintain, like new healthy habits or keeping a solid and healthy connection to your intuition, gets thrown out because you're just trying to live through all that pressure.

In this Aquarian Age, with all of the technology present in our everyday lives, we are chronically stressed-out. We process an exorbitant amount of information each day. Our nervous systems are under pressure with all this information, and many of us don't realize that, just like our technology, we need to upgrade our systems—our minds and our bodies—to manage the amount of stress we're under and to handle more of what we want in life.

When we continue to operate from a stressed-out place, wanting everything out of life but not able to handle it all, it can get straight-up frustrating. You can't keep up with what's already on your plate, let alone any of the new dreams you want to manifest. Think about it: if you're already dropping balls, losing mental focus, or getting into the bad-habit trap, adding more to your schedule—whether it's more clients for your business, a new relationship, or a big, new home—would probably push you over the edge.

This is why stress management is our first pillar—because everything is built upon how you can handle the tension that life is going to throw your way. Your system needs tools and practices to keep up with the amount of pressure it's facing. Stress is always going to happen, but you can learn how to manage it.

These morning rituals were created to help you manage your stress by reducing doubt, fear, anxiety, comparison, and judgment of yourself and others. They'll also help you release control by surrendering to the universe. Do you feel like you can breathe a little easier now?

After diving into one of these stress busters, you will be looking at yourself in the mirror and saying, "Who am I?" Answer: "Different, better, and I like what I see."

RITUAL 1 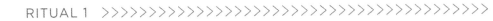 >>>

Natural Xanax
Reducing Fear and Anxiety

15-25 MINUTES

Living with anxiety is like driving an old, beat-up car: it will technically move you forward, but it's not a fun or easy ride, will break down often, and will drain your money and time.

Unfortunately, anxiety is an epidemic in today's fast-paced world. According to the World Health Organization (WHO), one in thirteen people globally suffers from this condition, making it the most common mental health disorder.[4] If you're prone to anxiety, you'll know that it's closely linked to stress—when you're under a lot of pressure at work or in your personal life, it can make anxiety symptoms even worse. But there's good news: a lot can be done to soothe an anxious mind. Research shows yoga and meditation can be helpful in treating anxiety, and a few small studies indicate that Kundalini yoga specifically may help support people with a formal diagnosis of general anxiety disorder.[5]

We curated this ritual to help you break free from the chains of anxiety. Releasing fear and anxiety will free you and allow you to actually live, versus struggling to get through the day. (Because that's what you're here for, right?) By releasing your own fear and anxiety, you not only bring peace to yourself, but you also contribute to improving the mental health crisis on the planet and help elevate the globe big time! Day one of forty days starts today!

> 66 99
>
> I USED TO WORRY ABOUT EVERYTHING, AND TO NUMB THAT ENERGY INSIDE ME, I WOULD GET DRUNK SO I COULD FORGET ABOUT IT ALL. BUT THAT JUST MADE THE ANXIETY SO MUCH WORSE IN THE LONG RUN. **I STARTED TO REALIZE THAT THERE HAD TO BE A BETTER WAY, AND I COMMITTED TO PRACTICING THE TOOLS IN THIS RITUAL.** THEN ONE NIGHT, WHEN I WAS OUT IN HOLLYWOOD AT 2:00 A.M. (YET AGAIN), I LOOKED IN THE MIRROR, AND A VOICE CAME THROUGH. IT SAID: 'YOU'RE BETTER THAN THIS, BRITT, AND YOU HAVE A LOT TO OFFER YOURSELF AND THE WORLD.' IT HIT ME HARD, AND I JUST GOT IT. I NEVER TOUCHED DRUGS AGAIN AND HAVEN'T BEEN DRUNK SINCE, AND MY MIND IS NOW ENTIRELY DIFFERENT. MY THOUGHTS DON'T RACE, MY MIND FEELS CLEAR, MY AWARENESS IS HEIGHTENED, AND INTUITIVE MESSAGES COME THROUGH. **I SET MYSELF FREE FROM MY ANXIETY AND SELF-DESTRUCTIVE HABITS THROUGH THE PRACTICES IN THIS RITUAL.**
>
> —*Britt*

Gather

- Yoga mat, meditation cushion, or chair.

- Amethyst crystal. Put your favorite amethyst crystal in your lap to help calm your nervous system and encourage logical thinking.

- Bergamot oil. Studies show this refreshing citrus oil may help relieve anxiety and improve mood.[6] Inhale the aroma two or three times before starting the ritual.

- Journal and pen.

- Glass of water. Drink a glass of water before this ritual and another glass after you finish the Natural Xanax Elixir at the end. It's important to stay hydrated all day, as dehydration has been linked to anxiety.[7]

- Ingredients for Natural Xanax Elixir.

Many studies link alcohol and caffeine with anxiety, so we recommend curbing the coffee and happy hours as much as possible for this forty-day ritual protocol.

Tune In

Come down onto your mat, sitting in a cross-legged position. Alternatively, you can sit in a chair with shoes off and both feet flat on the ground. Rub your palms together and bring them into your heart center in a prayer position. Begin your ritual by tuning in with the "Adi Mantra"—"Ong Namo Guroo Dayv Namo"—three times.

Mantra

Play the "33rd Pauri for Negativity and to Dissolve the Ego" during the breath and warm-up portions of the ritual. We love Snatam Kaur's version on the album *Meditation of the Soul: 11 Recitations of the Pauris of Jap Ji*. You can find it on the Spotify playlist, "Good Morning Intentions," we made to accompany this book!

Breathwork

Stay seated and get ready to do some breathwork to alleviate stress! This one literally washes the stress from your body and your aura, and fills you with calm, quiet, balance, and *prana*—life- force energy that flows through the body.[8] It's a very powerful technique to release anxiety.

Posture. Get comfortable in a cross-legged position with a straight spine, chin tucked slightly in, and chest lifted.

Mudra. Place your hands in Gyan Mudra, with the tips of the thumbs and index fingers touching and the rest of the fingers out straight, or any other comfortable, meditative mudra.

Eyes. Close your eyes and concentrate on your breath.

Breath. Inhale through your nose in eight equal breaths. Exhale through your nose in one deep and powerful breath.

Time. Continue repeating this breath pattern for three minutes.

To end. Inhale deeply and hold the breath for five to ten seconds. Exhale. Inhale deeply and hold the breath for fifteen to twenty seconds while rolling your shoulders forward. Exhale powerfully. Inhale deeply and hold the breath for fifteen to twenty seconds and roll the shoulders forward as fast as you can. Exhale and relax.

Warm-Up

Start by calming your nervous system with Cat-Cow. The Cat-Cow posture activates the spine—home to thirty-one pairs of nerves!—and balances the parasympathetic and sympathetic nervous systems, which allows us to handle stress with grace instead of fear and anxiety.

To begin, come onto your hands and knees. Your hands should be shoulder-width apart with fingers pointing forward. Make sure your knees are directly below your hips. Inhale and tilt your pelvis forward, arching the spine down, expanding the belly out, and stretching the head and neck up and back. Then exhale and tilt your pelvis the opposite way, arching the spine up and bringing the chin to the chest, contracting the belly into the spine. Make the motion very smooth and feel free to speed it up if you can. (In the Kundalini yoga practice, Cat-Cow is a rapid movement.) Close your eyes to go within and turn your gaze in and up so you're looking toward the point in between your eyebrows, which helps calm the mind. Continue for two minutes.

Meditation

Now come into the Kundalini Meditation to Tranquilize the Mind.[9]

Posture. Sit in Easy Pose (a cross-legged position) with a straight spine, your chin tucked slightly in a light "Neck Lock." You'll know you've done it correctly if you feel a little pressure at the back of the neck.

Mudra. The hand position is called "the mudra which pleases the mind." Buddha gave it to his disciples for control of the mind. With your elbows bent, bring your hands up to meet in front of your body at the level of the heart. Your elbows are held up almost to the level of the hands. Bend the Jupiter (index) fingers of each hand in toward your palms, and press the two Jupiter fingers together along the second joint. The Saturn (middle) fingers are extended and meet at the fingertips. The other fingers are curled into your hands. The thumb tips are joined and pointing toward your body. Hold the mudra parallel to the ground about four inches from your body with the extended fingers pointing away from your chest.

Eyes. Focus on the tip of your nose.

Breath + Mantra. Inhale completely and hold the breath while repeating the mantra "Saa Taa Naa Maa" eleven to twenty-one times. Exhale, hold the breath out, and repeat the mantra an equal number of times.

Time. Continue for three minutes.

Listen to the sound of the mantra and vibrate with it. Really feel into the mantra and be present with it. Don't just say it to say it; feel the sound running through you and embody it. You will get better and better at this the more you practice.

To end. Inhale deeply, suspend the breath, and exhale. Repeat one more time. Relax.

Seal your practice with Sat Naam. Bring your hands together in Prayer Pose in front of your heart. Inhale deeply and either chant or say out loud "Sat Naam," which means "truth is my essence."

Journal

Time for a brain dump! Write down two to five sources of fear and anxiety you are ready to release right now. It could be something about a current situation, a past trauma, or anything else that's bringing up fear and anxiety for you right now. At the bottom, write: "Thank you, I release you." (To make this exercise extra powerful, burn your list! Just be sure to do it safely.)

Affirmation

After the meditation, sit in silence and listen to anything that comes through. Then, repeat one of these affirmations at least once or create your own. They're most powerful when you say them out loud, and they've brought us and many others lots of peace.

In this moment, I choose to release the past, enjoy the moment, and look forward to all the amazing things to come.

I am safe.

I am supported.

I am improving.

My dominant intent is to feel good.

I attract peace and grace.

Everything that needs to get done today will get done.

I am at peace in the present moment.

Visualization

Visualize what your life would look like without fear and anxiety. What would be different? What would you be doing? How would things change? What would you feel, wear, be around, and so forth?

Nourishment

After your visualization, slowly make your way to the kitchen to mindfully prepare the Natural Xanax Elixir. This soothing elixir is rich in probiotics and magnesium, both of which can help improve anxiety. You can enjoy this elixir up to twice a day—it's a great substitute for coffee (or even a p.m. glass of wine!).

NATURAL XANAX ELIXIR

Prep time: 2 minutes
Makes 1 serving

1 cup spring water

Magnesium tea (for example the Calm brand) or magnesium powder

1 cup kombucha of your choice—one with turmeric, ginger, or lavender is great

Lemon juice to taste

>> Steep the magnesium tea or mix the powder in water. Combine all ingredients. Pour over ice, or if you want to enjoy it hot, heat up the whole thing. Enjoy!

Another nutrition note is to pay attention to how you feel when you eat meat today. If you notice anxiety afterward, it could be because the energies of anxiety and fear are present in animals before they are killed—especially in factory-farming situations. (We know, it's a little intense to hear, but we want you to be aware of that energy transfer.) If this resonates with you, consider giving up meat for at least forty days and see how it affects your anxiety.

MAKE IT YOUR INTENTION TODAY TO FEEL GOOD, HAVE FUN, AND BRING MORE JOY INTO THE PRESENT MOMENT NO MATTER WHAT YOU'RE DOING! **YOU DESERVE IT.** WE LOVE YOU AND HOPE YOU HAVE THE BEST DAY.

—XO, B+T

RITUAL 2 >>>

Comparison Detox
Stop Comparing to Others and Step into Greatness

20–40 MINUTES

Detoxing from comparison is like defriending the quintessential mean girl in high school. She's not your BFF. When you compare yourself to others, you shift into the low-vibration emotions of lack, separation, fear, and worry. This has a serious impact on your self-esteem and self-worth, as it leaves you feeling insecure. Thanks to social media—and the fact that we're faced with other people's highlight reels day in and day out—comparison truly has become an epidemic. So many struggle to manifest their dreams because they're wasting their energy on comparison—focusing on what they don't have and feeling like crap about it. They don't believe they deserve everything they want to magnetize, which makes it very difficult to be in the energy of manifestation. We created this ritual to help you heal these patterns and beliefs and step into your greatness...like, now. When you're not comparing yourself to others, you're free to celebrate the things that make *you* special and get back to feeling good. We love you, you are worthy, you're welcome!

> ❝❞
>
> I USED TO COMPARE MYSELF TO OTHERS WITHOUT EVEN REALIZING IT. MY SENSE OF SELF-WORTH WAS BASED ON GETTING THE BEST GRADES, NOT MISSING A DAY OF SCHOOL, GETTING THE BEST PART IN THE SCHOOL PLAY...AND IT WENT ON. BUT THROUGH THESE PRACTICES, **I REALIZED THAT I WASN'T DEFINED BY MY ACHIEVEMENTS. KUNDALINI YOGA HELPED ME MOVE A LOT OF ENERGY, AND I WAS ABLE TO MAKE FRIENDS WITH MY EGO.** I STARTED TO HAVE MORE COMPASSION FOR OTHERS AND NO LONGER CARED ABOUT PROVING MYSELF. MY NEW WAY OF MEASURING MYSELF WAS AND STILL IS, "AM I HAPPY?" INSTEAD OF, "AM I DOING BETTER THAN HARRY, DICK, AND SALLY?" ALL OF A SUDDEN, I WANTED HARRY, DICK, AND SALLY AND *EVERYONE* (INCLUDING MYSELF!) TO HAVE EVERYTHING THEY EVER WANTED. **IT WAS SUCH A HEALING JOURNEY, WHICH IS WHY I'M SO EXCITED FOR YOU TO EXPERIENCE THIS!**
>
> —*Britt*

Gather

- Yoga mat, meditation cushion, or chair.

- Angelite, green aventurine, or labradorite crystals. Hold one in your hands to promote a sense of security while you do the affirmations and visualization in this ritual.

- Sandalwood and jasmine oils. Melt your insecurities away by blending sixteen drops of sandalwood oil and four drops of jasmine oil in an essential-oil diffuser. You can also place four drops of sandalwood oil and one drop of jasmine into almond oil and rub the mixture onto your hands and arms before you begin.

- Journal and pen.

- Ingredients for Greatness Green Juice.

Mantra

Play the "Kundalini Mantra for Self-Esteem and Confidence" during your journaling session, warm-up, and meditation. This is known to pack a one-two punch, using both the English and the Gurmukhi translations of the mantra on most tracks. We love the one by Bachan Kaur titled "Bountiful, Blissful, Beautiful." You can find it on the Spotify playlist we made to accompany this book!

The Gurmukhi part of the mantra is from *Anand Sahib: The Song of Bliss*. It transports the soul into a state of bliss to aid you in connecting with the flow of Spirit.

Journal

List anything or anyone you are comparing yourself to today, and write down what you are saying to yourself as a result, such as, "You are not good enough," "You are not successful enough," and so on. Next to each statement, write whether or not it is true, kind, or necessary. Then come up with a truer, kinder, more helpful statement you can use whenever those thoughts come up. Practice pivoting your thoughts to the ones that are true, kind, and necessary. Paired with breathwork and meditation, this mind-set work will bring you the confidence you deserve!

Tune In

Come down onto your mat, sitting in a cross-legged position. Alternatively, you can sit in a chair with shoes off and both feet flat on the ground. Rub your palms together and bring them into your heart center in a prayer position. Begin your ritual by tuning in with the "Adi Mantra"—"Ong Namo Guroo Dayv Namo"—three times.

Warm-Up

Spinal Twists open up the heart and awaken the spine. This movement will get your energy flowing toward compassion instead of comparison.

Come to sitting on your heels in Rock Pose. Place your hands on your shoulders, your four fingers in front of your shoulders, and your thumbs in back. Your arms and elbows are parallel to the ground. (If this pose is too difficult, you can sit in a cross-legged position, or stand up with your feet shoulders-width apart.)

Inhale, expanding your stomach out, twisting your head and torso as far to the left as you can go. Then exhale, contract the stomach in, and twist your head and body as far to the right as you can go. Continue this movement back and forth for one to two minutes with your eyes closed, looking up between your brows to your third-eye point.

To end, come to the center, inhale deeply, and hold the breath as long as you can. Exhale fully to relax your arms down. Feel the energy circulating through your body and around your heart center.

Meditation

This three-part meditation, titled Let the Self Take Care of Things, was created to change your energetic frequency to allow in more compassion.[10] It will aid you in releasing the comparison game—the judgment of yourself and others—and in developing the self-love you need so you aren't looking outside of yourself for validation. Your soul knows how to take care of you if you just let it, and when it does, you will know you've got all you need and you're perfect as you are. The key is to find your divine self within yourself and then see what comes to you.

Choose to do the first two parts for three minutes or eleven minutes. If you do parts 1 and 2 for three minutes, do part 3 for one minute. If you do parts 1 and 2 for eleven minutes, do part 3 for three minutes.

PART 1

Posture. Sit up straight in a cross-legged position.

Mudra. Hold your hands together in Sarab Gyan Mudra in front of the heart. Begin by interlacing your fingers, then extend the index fingers up, pressing the palms and index fingers very tightly together, thumbs crossed.

Eyes. The eyes are closed.

Breath. With long, deep breathing, meditate on your breath, inhaling and exhaling so deeply and completely that you can hear your own breath. Continue for three or eleven minutes.

PART 2

Posture + Mudra + Eyes. Same as part 1.

Music. Listen to "Sat Narayan Wahe Guru" by Mata Mandir Singh. (You can find it on the Spotify playlist we made to accompany this book!)

Breath. Continue long, deep breathing in rhythm with the mantra. Inhale during one complete sound cycle (two repetitions of the mantra, about twenty seconds) and exhale during one complete sound cycle (two repetitions of the mantra, about twenty seconds). Carry on for three or eleven minutes.

PART 3

Posture + Mudra + Eyes. Same as parts 1 and 2.

Breath. Do a powerful Breath of Fire: Inhale and exhale, equal in strength and length, through the nose. Allow the navel point (the energy center located two to three inches below the belly button) to move with the breath, expanding on the inhale, contracting on the exhale. Speed up this movement and begin to pump the navel point. Continue for one to three minutes, doing your best during the last minute. Note: If you're on the first three days of your moon cycle or you're pregnant, do long, deep breathing instead.

To end. Inhale deeply, suspend the breath, and exhale. Repeat one more time. Relax.

Seal your practice with Sat Naam. Bring your hands together in Prayer Pose in front of your heart. Inhale deeply and either chant or say out loud "Sat Naam," which means "truth is my essence."

Affirmation

After the meditation, sit in silence and listen to anything that comes through. Then, repeat the following affirmation at least five times. It's most powerful when you say it out loud and put it into your aura using the throat chakra. Feel free to say this mantra whenever you find yourself in comparison mode—it will help shift and pivot your thoughts and vibration in those moments.

I cannot be compared to anyone or anything. I am uniquely me for a divine purpose and I trust in my greatness.

Visualization

Visualize yourself in front of you. Send yourself love and feel it pouring over you in a waterfall of pink healing light.

Next, visualize anyone you compare yourself to or feel negative energy toward. See them as a reflection of you—the beauty you see in them is also in you! Send that same love and pink healing light to each of them.

Lastly, picture yourself sending that love and healing pink light to everyone you come into contact with. Take a minute to imagine what the world would look like if everyone released competition and came together in unity and compassion. How would everyone treat each other? How would that feel? What would it look like if you engaged in this way?

Self-Care

Positive self-talk is an act of self-love. It's so important to overcome insecurities that cause us to compare ourselves, and so it's time to talk yourself up—think of this as your daily pep talk!

Before you leave your mat, say three nice things to yourself out loud or in your head. Examples: "You are incredibly radiant and bright. You light up the whole room. You are brilliant, beautiful, and such a badass!"

If you feel insecure about something specific, say something nice about that part of you or take an inspired action to give yourself love. For example, if you're self-conscious about the way your hands look (like Britt!), you could give yourself a hand massage with your favorite oil. Or if you have insecurities about your abs (like Tara!), say nice things to your stomach, send it love, and hold it. It's all about sending love to the parts of you that need it the most.

Nourishment

To really feel good and start the day with tons of love for yourself, drink this super simple Greatness Green Juice! Within forty days your skin, hair, and inner organs will be thanking you big time.

GREATNESS GREEN JUICE

Prep time: 5 minutes
Makes 1 serving

1 large apple (Pink Lady recommended)

1 bunch celery

1 lemon

1-inch piece fresh ginger, peeled

5 fresh mint leaves

¼ bunch cilantro

>> Place all the ingredients in a high-speed juicer. You can also use a blender and strain the pulp using cheesecloth or a strainer. Pour into a glass and enjoy right away! If you are taking it to go, put it in a fun reusable cup for the road.

YOU'VE GOT THIS DAY! THE MORE YOU FOCUS ON YOU AND SHINE YOUR LIGHT OUT, THE BETTER YOU'LL FEEL—PROMISE. WE ARE BLINDED BY YOUR GREATNESS AND SO GRATEFUL YOU EXIST.

—XO, B+T

RITUAL 3 >>>

Let the Universe Take the Wheel
Reverse Control

25-30 MINUTES

Pop quiz! Do you try to control every outcome in your life? Do you have a hard time letting things go? Do you push to make things happen instead of attracting opportunities to you? Do you have high expectations for yourself and others—and if your expectations aren't met, do you blame everyone else for not living up to your vision of how things should have gone? If you answered yes to any of these questions, you likely need a control intervention. Lucky for you, we have a morning ritual for that!

Control is a hassle birthed from the ego. It's the feeling of holding on so tight to a vision, person, place, or thing that there's no room for flexibility or growth. Instead, the opposite happens. You hold on so tight that whatever you're gripping begins to contract. In this situation, your ego gets what it wants—for you to be in the same place you're in now because it's safer than the unknown. The direct opposite of control is surrender, letting go of your expectations, dropping your ego's agenda, taking responsibility for your emotions, and trusting something bigger than yourself to be your guide. This control-intervention ritual is designed to adjust your compass from the safety of control to the beauty of surrender.

"

I HAD TO UNKNOT A LOT OF CONTROL ISSUES IN MY OWN LIFE. IT WAS HARD FOR ME TO ACCEPT THAT LIFE COULD FLOW IN A BIGGER AND MORE BEAUTIFUL WAY THAN MY MIND COULD ENVISION. IN MY RELATIONSHIPS, I WOULD PROJECT HOW I THOUGHT SOMEONE SHOULD ACT AND RESPOND OUT OF FEAR AND INSECURITY. IN MY CAREER, I MET CHANGE WITH HEAVY RESISTANCE SO I DIDN'T HAVE TO FEEL UNCOMFORTABLE OR UNSAFE. BUT ALL THIS DID WAS KEEP ME IN THE SAFE ZONE, AND IT PRODUCED A LOT OF FRUSTRATION BECAUSE I WASN'T LETTING MYSELF EXPAND. **WHEN I LEARNED TO SURRENDER TO THE FLOW OF MY LIFE AND REALIZED MY CONTROL WAS REALLY JUST A WAY OF AVOIDING MY OWN INNER GROWTH, EVERYTHING CHANGED.** ELEVATE THE GLOBE WAS DELIVERED TO BRITT AND ME THROUGH THIS SURRENDER. I GAVE MYSELF OVER TO THE UNIVERSE TO BE OF SERVICE TO MYSELF AND OTHERS, AND I FOLLOWED THE PATH THAT SHOWED UP THROUGH CONSTANT SURRENDER EACH DAY. IT CHANGED MY LIFE. THIS MORNING RITUAL WILL HELP YOU PRACTICE KEEPING A LOOSE GRIP AND LETTING LIFE FLOW THROUGH YOU. THINK OF IT AS HOLDING HANDS WITH THE UNIVERSE.

—Tara

Gather

- Yoga mat, meditation cushion, or chair.

- Lapis lazuli crystal. Hold it during your meditation or wear it as a piece of jewelry to cleanse your thoughts and surrender to higher spiritual realms.

- Lavender oil. Place a few drops with a carrier oil like almond oil on your wrists and behind your ears before your morning ritual—it can help calm and relax your mind and body.

- Your calendar, a journal, and a pen.

- Melon.

Tune In

Come down onto your mat, sitting in a cross-legged position. Alternatively, you can sit in a chair with shoes off and both feet flat on the ground. Rub your palms together and bring them into your heart center in a prayer position. Begin your ritual by tuning in with the "Adi Mantra"—"Ong Namo Guroo Dayv Namo"—three times.

Mantra

Play the mantra "Ek Ong Kaar Satgur Parsaad, Satgur Parsaad, Ek Ong Kaar" as you practice this ritual's warm-up and meditation. (We love the version "Expand into Intuitive Knowing [Ek Ong Kar Sat Gur Prasad]" by Jai-Jagdeesh.) This mantra is incredibly powerful and amps up your positivity and manifestation powers, helping you loosen the tight grip you have on your life so you can surrender and know you're exactly where you're meant to be. When played—and especially when chanted out loud—it can bring you great awareness, intuitive ability, and remove all obstacles in your way. All the things you need to go from control to surrender!

Warm-Up

Come to a kneeling position on your knees with your bum on your heels for Sitting Bends. Interlace your fingers behind your neck, dropping your shoulders down and pulling your elbows back. Inhale, sitting tall, and as you exhale, bend your body forward, bringing your forehead to the ground. Move from the hips to push yourself back up on the inhale. Continue this movement for one to three minutes.

If sitting on your heels doesn't feel good, you can also come into Easy Pose (a cross-legged position) and bend forward from the waist, touching your forehead to the ground. If you can't get your forehead to touch the ground, that's okay—just go as far as you can.

To end, deeply inhale with your fingers still interlaced behind your neck and elbows back. Hold the breath for as long as you can, then exhale and relax your body.

Meditation

This meditation, Surrender to Your Intuition, will help you increase the flow of breath (prana) to the crown chakra.[11] When it's balanced and strong, this chakra allows you to surrender to the cosmic flow and gives you guidance so you don't need to control anything—instead, you're guided to everything you need. The placement of your arms will release a powerful stimulant to the pineal and pituitary glands, which will result in an increase in intuition. This one will take practice to perfect—but it'll get easier over time!

Posture. Sit in Easy Pose (a cross-legged position), with your chin pulled down and back in a light Neck Lock. Extend your arms up over your head in a circular arc (like a ballerina pose) so the palms and fingers of each hand face down about six to eight inches over the crown of your head. The hands are separated by about twelve inches overhead and the thumbs separate from the fingers and hang loosely.

Breath. Breathe in a three-part pattern:

1. Inhale in eight equal breaths.

2. Exhale completely in eight equal breaths.

3. Hold the breath out for a count of sixteen in the same rhythm.

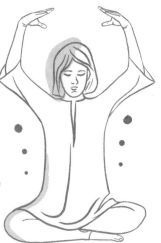

Mantra. Mentally repeat the mantra "Saa Taa Naa Maa" eight times with each full cycle of the breathwork—one syllable for every breath.

Eyes. Fix your eyes one-tenth open so they're almost closed, but allow a sliver of light in.

Time. Continue for eleven minutes, with the option to increase to twenty-two minutes and slowly build up to thirty-one minutes.

To end. Inhale deeply, raise your arms up higher over your head, and stretch your arms up and backward as far as you can. Drop your head back and look up to the sky. Stretch with all your strength to extend the lower back and the neck. Then exhale and let the arms down. Then swing your arms back up and repeat this final breath two more times. Rest for a few moments in a seated position.

Seal your practice with Sat Naam. Bring your hands together in Prayer Pose in front of your heart. Inhale deeply and either chant or say out loud "Sat Naam," which means "truth is my essence."

Watch the thoughts and emotions that come up as you keep your arms overhead— what stories are playing out in this meditation that you're carrying out into the rest of your life? Are you focusing on how hard it is? Do you want to give up? Are you getting angry or frustrated? Do you wish things were different? See if you can surrender into the arm placement, even if it's uncomfortable. Focus on the breath and the mantra to carry you through.

Journal

Look at your schedule for today and identify situations and interactions where you can practice releasing control and being more flexible. Write down ways you can surrender more into being guided by the universe, wherever the day may bring you.

Affirmation

To complete your ritual, remain in a seated position with your palms facing up. Then, recite this affirmation:

> *Universe, I surrender to your guidance today. I will listen to and follow my impulses to go wherever you would have me go and say whatever you would have me say today.*

This affirmation is the ultimate statement to yourself and the universe that you're ready to release control and are open to being guided by something bigger than yourself. Each morning, allow your ego to step aside so your higher self can come through and be of service to you and everyone you come in contact with.

Feel yourself commit to showing up this way today. It's safe to loosen your grip and be guided all day long!

Nourishment

For the forty days of your control intervention ritual, we recommend eating melon for breakfast. Not only is it used to reduce inflammation—a major side effect of stress—but spiritually speaking, it helps us magnetize what we need and trust that it will arrive.[12]

> **66 99**
>
> YOU'RE RELEASING AND RELAXING AND BECOMING MORE OF THAT BEAUTIFUL *YOU* IN EVERY MOMENT OF EACH DAY. WE LOVE HOW YOU'RE SHOWING UP TO BE OF SERVICE AND LETTING THE NEED TO CONTROL SLIP AWAY. YOU'VE GOT THIS, YOU BEAUTIFUL BEAM OF LIGHT, AND WE LOVE YOU!
>
> *—Sat Naam, B+T*

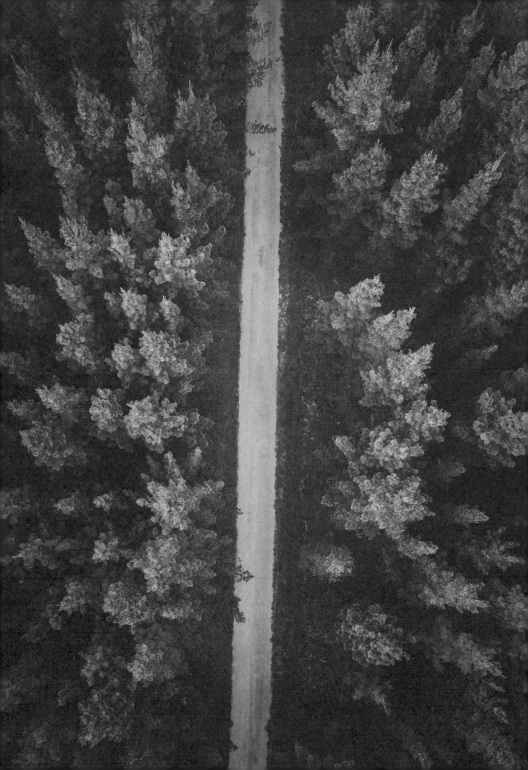

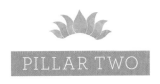

Mind-Set

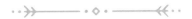

The Universal Law of Mentalism states that everything is mental; the universe is a mental creation of the all. If you aren't manifesting the career, money, relationships, or body you want, there may be an untrue story, a deep wound that needs healing, a limiting belief, or negative self-talk getting in the way of your intentions—and you might not even be aware of it. If you're facing any external challenges that are out of your control, like an illness or financial hardship, these stories can make it even harder to call in what you really want. That's why mind-set training is the second pillar of the Elevate the Globe lifestyle. See, when your mind-set is distorted, like a compass that's off-kilter, everything in your reality will match that imbalanced energy. When this happens, you'll inevitably end up at some less-than-desirable destinations.

The Universal Law of Mentalism states that everything we experience in the external world starts in the mind—particularly the subconscious and unconscious mind, which drive our habits. In other words, perception is reality: things are how you think they are, and you get what you expect. But thoughts in our subconscious and unconscious are *not* conscious to us, so we have no idea why the F we aren't getting where we want to go. This is why you may have an area of your life where you want one thing, but you keep getting something else. You might *think* you want a relationship, but you keep going on bad dates. Or maybe you have the desire to lose weight, stop gossiping, have $100K in your bank account, or start pursuing your passions, but you continuously attract the opposite of that.

If this is where you are right now, don't get down on yourself! Trust us, we've been there. But through our journey, we figured out that the key is to pair mind-set training and high-level mindfulness techniques with the potent energy work of Kundalini yoga. This combination makes you an unstoppable force in all areas of life. It shifts the subconscious patterns that are holding you back, putting your mind back into balance so it's easy to follow the map to your wildest dreams. This is a journey that takes commitment, but ultimately, you'll feel really good about yourself, trust your path completely, be guided by your higher self, and become more and more aligned with your truth, confidence, and gifts. Having a limitless, love-based mind-set focused on awareness and healing has allowed us to shift our experience in the world, step into our power and abundance, and really feel happiness from living our purpose and doing what we love.

We created the rituals in this section to heal your dominant thoughts and shift your emotions into a higher frequency—particularly when it comes to money and confidence, which are two things that our community asks us about the most. Your mind-set can also impact the way you look on the outside, so we've included a morning practice for radiance in this section too! When you practice one of these rituals for forty days, you can expect to see a change in the way you feel, and that will eventually be reflected in your outer reality. Mind-set training is all about learning how to live in the neutral mind—not reacting to life but being proactive and coming from a place of love and compassion. How great does that sound?

The Gold Rush
Prosperity

20-25 MINUTES

Often, what's keeping you from experiencing a gold rush of prosperity in your own life comes down to learned beliefs you've picked up from your experiences. Here's the thing: if you're not happy with how these beliefs have shaped your reality, then it's time to readjust your thinking and clear out those subconscious ideas that are keeping you from seeing and receiving all the "gold" that's available to you. Strip everything back to your Sat Naam, your truth, and embody prosperity in all areas of life. Everything else is just dirt in the pan clouding your vision.

We curated this ritual to help you align your mind-set to manifest great wealth—not just when it comes to money (although that's definitely a big part of it!), but also in terms of the things money can't buy, such as vibrant health, abundant friendships, and a fulfilling love life. Commit to this ritual for forty days for maximum benefits.

Gather

- Yoga mat, meditation cushion, or chair.
- Pyrite crystal. Keep pyrite nearby during this ritual to energetically attune yourself to a wealth frequency.

- Sweet basil oil. Breathe it in or blend it with almond oil and dab it on your pulse points before you begin, as this essential oil is associated with money and abundance.

- Journal and pen.

- Ingredients for Yogi Tea or a Yogi Tea-brand tea bag.

Assemble the ingredients for this ritual's Yogi Tea recipe the night before. Then warm them on the stove before your practice so your tea will be ready for you when you're done!

Tune In

Come down onto your mat, sitting in a cross-legged position. Alternatively, you can sit in a chair with shoes off and both feet flat on the ground. Rub your palms together and bring them to your heart center in a prayer position. Begin your ritual by tuning in with the "Adi Mantra"—"Ong Namo Guroo Dayv Namo"—three times.

Mantra

Play the "25th Pauri for Prosperity" during the breath and warm-up portions of the ritual. For extra prosperity, feel free to play it any other time throughout the day and while you sleep at night. (We love Snatam Kaur's version on the album *Meditation of the Soul: 11 Recitations of the Pauris of Jap Ji*. You can find it on the Spotify playlist that accompanies this book.)

Breathwork

Ego Eradicator with Breath of Fire opens the lungs, consolidates the magnetic field, and brings the brain hemispheres to a state of alertness. This allows you to be open andmagnetize things to you from a high frequency—money receptive, and toincluded!

Posture. This exercise can be done in Easy Pose (sitting in a cross-legged position) or Rock Pose (in a kneeling position with your bum resting on your heels). Raise your arms up and out to the sides in a V at a sixty-degree angle. Keep your elbows straight and your shoulders down. Pull your chin down and back so your spine is straight. Curl your fingertips onto the pads of the palms at the base of the fingers. Thumbs are stretched back, pointing toward each other.

Eyes. Eyes are closed.

Mental focus. Focus above the head.

Breath. Inhale and exhale, equal in strength and length, through the nose. Allow the navel point (the energy center located two to three inches below the belly button) to move with the breath, expanding on the inhale, contracting on the exhale. Speed up this movement and begin to pump the navel point. Note: If you're on the first three days of your moon cycle or you're pregnant, do long, deep breathing instead.

Time. Continue for one to three minutes.

To end. Inhale deeply and bring your arms overhead with the thumb tips touching. Open the other four fingers and stretch your arms up, then exhale and release your hands down.

Warm-Up

Spinal flexes cultivate a balanced root chakra, which is essential to attract and sustain wealth.

To begin, sit in Easy Pose (a cross-legged position) with your hands holding your ankles. Lightly pull on your ankles as you inhale, arching your spine forward and pulling your shoulders back. Exhale as you round out your spine and release it backward. Your head does not move, and your chin stays parallel to the ground. Concentrate on massaging the base of the spine into the ground, and continue this movement for three minutes.

This movement can also be performed sitting on your heels or in a chair, placing your hands on your knees.

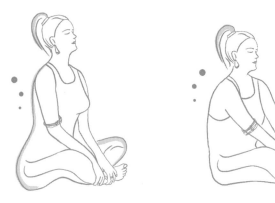

Meditation

This is a powerful prosperity meditation that has a limit of practicing eleven minutes a day because the wisdom of Kundalini yoga states that any more than that would be greedy.[13] What you're doing in this meditation is stimulating the mind (which creates your reality), the moon center (which rules your emotions that manifest your reality), and your Jupiter fingers (the planet of luck and expansion), so wealth manifests easily.

Posture. Sit in Easy Pose, with your chin pulled down and back so your spine is straight. Elbows are by your sides, forearms angled up and outward with your fingers at the level of your throat. The exercise begins with the palms facing down.

Movement. When the palms face down, the sides of your Jupiter (index) fingers touch, and the thumbs cross below your hands, with the right thumb under the left and the wrists straight. Make note about your thumbs crossing this way as it is the key to the meditation. Now, alternately hit the opposite sides of your hands together so your palms face up. Your Mercury (pinky) fingers and moon mounds (located under the pinkies on the bottom of the palms) hit each other when the palms face up. As you complete both movements continuously, it will appear as though you're creating a circle with your hands in front of you.

Mantra. Chant "Har" every time the sides of your hands hit each other. (To create the "r" sound, flick the tongue against the upper palate behind the front teeth.) Chant continuously from the navel, using the tip of your tongue to hit the roof of your mouth with every recitation. You can chant along with the "Tantric Har" track by White Sun found on the Spotify playlist that accompanies this book.

Eyes. Look at the tip of the nose, through eyes nine-tenths of the way closed.

Time. Continue for three to eleven minutes.

Chant with conviction and power from your navel point (the energy center located two to three inches below the belly button). Command the mantra through your body and strike the hands together with meaning. It's important to note that eleven minutes is the maximum amount of time given to practice this meditation each day—any more would be greedy because of its power!

To end. Inhale with your palms facing up to receive. Exhale and relax your hands down.

Seal your practice with Sat Naam. Bring your hands together in Prayer Pose in front of your heart. Inhale deeply and either chant or say out loud "Sat Naam," which means "truth is my essence."

Journal

Write down two to five things you are thankful for in regard to prosperity *right now*—no matter what your present circumstances are. It can be something as small as the fact that you have clean water to drink or that the sun is shining. Whatever you choose, really feel into the energy of gratitude for each item on your list!

Affirmation

After the meditation, sit in silence and listen to anything that comes through. Then, repeat this affirmation, created by best-selling author and Law of Attraction teacher Bob Proctor, at least once. It's most powerful when you say it out loud, and it's brought us and many others great abundance.

> *I am so happy and grateful now that money flows to me in increasing quantities through multiple sources on a consistent basis.*

Visualization

Experiment with feeling the presence of both white and gold light after your meditation and visualize how you feel with new levels of prosperity. What does that look like for all of the senses?

Self-Care

Take a cold shower after your ritual—inspired by a Kundalini yoga practice called Ishnaan, it will wake up your nervous system, get your blood pumping, and set you up to slay the day! Prepare your body by massaging with oil or dry brushing, and then ease into the shower by massaging one limb at a time under the cold water, working up to putting your whole body in. Try to stay in the water for up to three minutes or until your body feels warm. If this is too intense for you, start by washing your hands, forearms, face, ears, and feet with cold water.

Nourishment

Whenever you go into a traditional Kundalini yoga studio, you'll smell freshly made Yogi Tea. It's especially powerful for grounding, which is vital when you're attracting abundance because being grounded is like giving Amazon.com your address so they know where to deliver your package.

Based on the knowledge of Ayurveda, Yogi Tea is traditionally thought to have the following benefits on the mind and body. It's traditionally made with dairy milk, but we substitute plant-based milk.

- Black pepper purifies the blood.
- Cinnamon strengthens the bones.
- Cardamom supports the colon.
- Cloves build the nervous system.
- Black tea (tiny amount) holds it all together.
- Coconut milk protects the colon.
- Ginger heals the digestive system.

We recommend making it fresh, but you can also buy the tea bags pre-made.

YOGI TEA

Prep time: 20–25 minutes
Makes 1 serving

10 ounces water (about 1 ¼ cups)

3 whole cloves

4 whole green cardamom pods, cracked

4 whole black peppercorns

½ stick cinnamon

2 slices fresh ginger, peeled

¼ teaspoon black tea

½ cup coconut or other nut milk

Maple syrup to taste (optional)

>> Bring the water to a boil and add the spices and ginger. Cover and boil 15 to 20 minutes, then add the black tea. Let sit for a few minutes, then add the coconut milk, and return to a boil. Don't let it boil over. When the mixture reaches a boil, remove immediately from the heat, strain, and sweeten with maple syrup, if desired.

66 99

YOU'VE DONE IT! GO FORTH IN YOUR DAY KNOWING THAT PROSPERITY IS YOUR BIRTHRIGHT; IT'S YOURS! YOU'RE BECOMING A MAGNET FOR ABUNDANCE TO COME TO YOU IN ALL ASPECTS OF YOUR LIFE, AND IT'S STARTING TO SHOW UP FOR YOU MORE AND MORE EVERY DAY. WOO-HOO!

—XO, B+T

Shield Your Power
Energetic Protection

25–30 MINUTES

Have you ever been in a situation that makes you feel drained, anxious, or just plain unhappy for no obvious reason? If so, you may be picking up on the energy of another person and that environment and taking it on yourself—something that's super common for those on the spiritual path.

In yogic philosophy, protecting your own energy is a matter of strengthening your circumvent force, or your aura. Your aura is like a bubble of light surrounding you—it's made up of energy from all of your chakras. Your aura is also affected by your mind-set—it's strengthened by all of your positive thoughts and weakened by your negativity. It both attracts things into your life and protects you from taking on others' vibratory frequencies. You arrived here on the planet with this built-in energetic shield, and it's your most powerful protection tool. When your aura is strong and radiant, negative thoughts, people, spirits, and energy can't touch you.

A few signs that your shield of protection could use some strength training are things like lacking clear boundaries with people, being unable to say no to them, and attracting negative people and painful events into your life. Frequently taking on other people's energy makes you feel extremely sensitive emotionally and affects your mind-set.

This morning ritual will help create a bubble of light around you so you can trust that you're safe and secure at all times. We're going to charge up your aura and fuel it with your own positivity because every thought you have and every action you take fortifies this protective shield around you.

Gather

- Yoga mat, meditation cushion, or chair.

- Obsidian or black tourmaline crystal. Obsidian can help you ground and release negativity, while black tourmaline is used for protection against psychic attacks. For best results, keep it by your mat during the ritual and then carry it with you all day!

- Frankincense oil. Put some in a diffuser to energetically protect and purify your space.

- Sage bundle, lighter, and shell or ceramic bowl.

- Holy basil tea bag.

Tune In

Come down onto your mat, sitting in a cross-legged position. Alternatively, you can sit in a chair with shoes off and both feet flat on the ground. Rub your palms together and bring them into your heart center in a prayer position. Begin your ritual by tuning in with the "Adi Mantra"—"Ong Namo Guroo Dayv Namo"—three times.

Mantra

Play the "Aad Guray Nameh" mantra while you practice the Shield Your Power ritual (described below). This sacred sound current has four lines: "Aad Guray Nameh / Jugaad Guray Nameh / Sat Guray Nameh / Siree Gurdayvay Nameh." It opens you up to guidance from the Divine and surrounds your aura with a protective shield. We love the version called "Aad Guray Nameh" by Snatam Kaur. (You can find it on the Spotify playlist we made to accompany this book!)

Chant the "Aad Guray Nameh" mantra three times, anytime you need a little extra energetic protection throughout your day. You can chant it before heading out the door, getting into the car, going into a meeting, or seeing a friend or family member. It can be used for any and all situations, to shield yourself and others.

Up your game. Chant this protective mantra around yourself in a circle for full auric protection.

Chant:

"Aad Guray Nameh" while focusing in front of you

"Jugaad Guray Nameh" as you bring your attention to your right side

"Sat Guray Nameh" while mentally focusing behind you

"Siree Gurdayvay Nameh" as you bring your attention to your left side

Warm-Up

Come up to a standing position for Archer Pose, an empowering posture that builds up that circumvent force around you—your auric field.

Spread your feet approximately two to three feet apart. Place your right foot forward and your left foot behind you and turned out to the left at a forty-five-degree angle. Root down through both legs. Bend the front knee until it is directly over the ankle. Keep the back leg straight. Feel a stretch between the two thighs and in front of the hip of the back leg.

Then, bring both arms parallel to the ground. Curl the fingers of both hands onto the palms, thumbs facing up. As if you're pulling back on a bow and arrow, extend your right arm out over your right knee.
Bend your left arm at the elbow and bring your left hand to your left shoulder.

Lengthen your spine, tuck your chin in, and open your chest. Breathe long and deep for one minute in this posture, staring out at the thumb in front of you. Then, switch sides and practice on the other side for one minute.

When you're finished, come down onto your mat in Easy Pose (a crossed-legged position).

Meditation

This Kundalini yoga practice is called the Chii-a Kriya.[14] This meditation is said to ward off negativity and surround you with protection from the six directions—north, south, east, west, up, and down. You have all your angles covered!

Posture. Sit in Easy Pose (a cross-legged position).

Mudra. Place your hands in Gyan Mudra by touching the tips of the thumbs and the tips of the Jupiter fingers (index fingers). The other fingers are relaxed.

Movement + Mantra. Keeping your hands in this mudra, close your eyes and move your arms in the following sequence:

1. Stretch your arms out to the sides with palms facing forward. Keep your elbows straight. Chant "Har." (To create the "r" sound, flick the tongue against the upper palate behind the front teeth.)

2. Without bringing your hands near your shoulders, move your hands directly in front of you with your palms down, elbows by your sides, and your forearms pointing straight out in front of your body. Chant "Haray." (Again, to create the "r" sound, flick the tongue against the upper palate behind the front teeth.)

3. Bring your hands up by your shoulders, palms facing out. Chant "Haree." (Here too, to create the "r" sound, flick the tongue against the upper palate behind the front teeth.)

4. Stretch your arms out to the sides again. Chant "Whaa."

5. Bring your arms directly to the front, palms down. Chant "Hay."

6. Bring your hands up near your shoulders. Chant "Guroo." (It's the same "r" sound here also: flick the tongue against the upper palate behind the front teeth.)

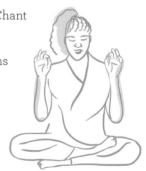

Chant strongly from your navel point (the energy center located two to three inches below the belly button).

Time. Continue for eleven minutes.

To end. With your arms in position 6, inhale and hold the breath for fifteen to twenty seconds. Squeeze your rib cage as you stretch your spine upward. Exhale. Repeat this sequence two more times. Bring your hands down onto your knees, palms facing up.

Seal your practice with Sat Naam. Bring your hands together in Prayer Pose in front of your heart. Inhale deeply and either chant or say out loud "Sat Naam," which means "truth is my essence."

Visualization

Picture a bright white light surrounding your entire body, emanating outward from you in all directions. Watch it begin to pulsate and get brighter and brighter, wider and wider. Now, send it out into the room and as far and wide as you can imagine. Feel your heart center open and send love into this white light in all directions. Breathe long and deep here for a few moments.

Affirmation

"I am" statements are incredibly powerful in situations when you're feeling vulnerable. Say this affirmation out loud now and keep it with you throughout your day so you can come back to it when you need a little protection. You can also use the protection mantra from this ritual—"Aad Guray Nameh"—when you need extra support.

I am surrounded by bright, white, radiant light and send out love in my every interaction. I am protected.

Feeling frightened or attacked by negative energies? When one person's negative thoughts are constantly directed toward someone else, it's called a psychic attack. To stop it and mirror the energy back to the person or spirit it originates from, powerfully chant this mantra only once.

Alahk Baabaa Siree Chand Dee Rakh

Again, it's important to only chant this mantra once per day and let it go—do not chant it over and over. If you repeat the mantra, you begin to psychically attack the person or spirit back, which then creates more of this back-and-forth.

Self-Care

Smudging yourself with sage is like taking an energetic shower. It's a ritual practice that goes back thousands of years and taps you into a long and deep spiritual line of history. Sage is used to purify the aura, cleanse negativity, and uplift the energy in a space. If you choose to use this tool, it's important to acknowledge and respect the indigenous people who place it at the center of their sacred ceremonies—perhaps even growing your own white sage or other herbs to burn, as this is the most sustainable, culturally sensitive way of adopting the practice.

You'll need a bundle of sage (or another herb of your choice), a lighter (we like to light ours on a gas stove burner), and a shell or ceramic bowl to catch any embers. Before you begin, state your intention. For example, "I ask the spirit of this sacred sage plant to come through and clear out all negativity around me. May anything that is not of love, light, and my highest good be washed away."

Light your sage and begin to move the bundle around your hands, cleansing them first. Then move up to the top of your head and begin to make your way down the front and back of your body until you get to your feet. Don't forget to pick up those feet and sage the bottoms of them—your energetic field goes all the way to and into the ground.

While you smudge yourself, you can chant the protection mantra "Aad Guray Nameh."

When finished, close the ritual by saying thank you to the sage, thank you to the Earth, and thank you to your spirit guides. Put out the burning edges of the sage in the ceramic bowl and dump the ashes outside in the dirt.

Nourishment

In the world of magic, it has long been believed that holy basil keeps unwanted spirits and negativity away. Before you head out for the day, head to the kitchen and make yourself a cup of holy basil tea. You can buy it in tea-bag form, which makes it easy to carry herbal protection with you everywhere.

> YOU ARE SO PROTECTED, AND WE'RE PROUD OF YOU FOR COMMITTING TO CLEANSING AND SAFEGUARDING YOUR ENERGY FIELD. NEGATIVITY CAN'T TOUCH YOU, GORGEOUS! YOUR SHIELD OF PROTECTION IS GETTING STRONGER EVERY SINGLE DAY. YOU'RE A WARRIOR AND WE LOVE YOU!
>
> —*XO B+T*

Shine Your Light
Self-Confidence and Worthiness

30-35 MINUTES

Confidence comes from a place of knowing exactly who you are, at the deepest core of you—at your truth. It doesn't come from what you think you should be or what someone else told you to be. It comes from experiencing yourself and accepting yourself fully. This is where the power of your confidence comes from: looking at all of your light and all of your shadows, and accepting them as part of who you are before deciding who you want to become.

Lack of self-confidence is a widespread energetic disease. It looks like not being able to trust your own opinions, constantly overthinking, being your own worst critic, being afraid to take on challenges, and dealing with frequent emotional turmoil and anxiety. All of these are symptoms of being too much in the mind and avoiding going within to look deeply into your soul.

But you're here to change all of this, so high freakin' five, my friend! Seriously, amazing job for showing up and getting to know yourself at a deep level so you can walk through your life standing tall—knowing exactly who you are so you can follow your dreams with confidence and know that you are beyond worthy of everything you attract into your life.

Stay open, be compassionate with yourself, and let this ritual guide you on your journey of self-discovery. We think you're really going to like what you see in yourself.

""

WHEN I THINK BACK TO WHEN I WAS YOUNGER, ONE OF THE MAIN THINGS THAT STANDS OUT IN MY MIND WAS THIS ONGOING STORY THAT I LACKED CONFIDENCE IN MYSELF. IT WAS SOMETHING I KNEW DEEPLY, MY PARENTS KNEW AND TALKED WITH ME ABOUT, AND ALL MY DANCE TEACHERS KNEW AND DISCUSSED WITH ME. IT FELT LIKE THIS HUGE ISSUE BECAUSE IT WAS. IT WOULD AFFECT WHAT I FELT LIKE I DESERVED—THE KINDS OF JOBS I'D APPLY FOR, THE PEOPLE I'D DATE, THE FRIENDS I'D MAKE. EVERY SINGLE THING IN MY LIFE WAS AFFECTED BY THIS LACK OF CONFIDENCE AND NOT FEELING WORTHY. **IT WASN'T UNTIL WELL INTO MY ADULT LIFE THAT I REALIZED MY LACK OF CONFIDENCE WAS DIRECTLY TIED TO MY LACK OF KNOWING MYSELF ON A DEEP LEVEL. MIND BLOWN!** THIS JOURNEY OF SELF-DISCOVERY STARTED WITH MY KUNDALINI YOGA PRACTICE, AND AS THE LAYERS OF ILLUSIONS PEELED AWAY—THE VERSIONS OF MYSELF I THOUGHT I SHOULD BE IN MY MIND—I STARTED TO NOTICE I FINALLY HAD MORE CONFIDENCE IN MYSELF. IT STILL GROWS EVERY SINGLE DAY. SO FOR ANYONE WHO HAS REALLY STRUGGLED WITH LACK OF CONFIDENCE AND FEELING UNWORTHY, I TOTALLY GET IT, AND I'M EXCITED FOR YOU TO EXPERIENCE THIS RITUAL TO GET TO KNOW YOURSELF ON A DEEPER LEVEL.

—Tara

Gather

- Yoga mat, meditation cushion, or chair.

- Carnelian crystal. This is a stone of courage, joy, and willpower that is great for building confidence and a sense of self-worth. Keep a carnelian stone next to your mat during your ritual and take it with you when you're in situations where you're communicating with others. It will help amplify the energy work you're doing within this morning practice.

- Bergamot oil. Place a couple of drops into a diffuser or blend it with almond oil and dab it behind your ears to help balance your mind and project positive, happy, and fun thoughts. It's easier to build confidence and worthiness in yourself when you don't take life too seriously and have fun!

- Journal and pen.

- Mint tea.

Tune In

Come down onto your mat, sitting in a cross-legged position. Alternatively, you can sit in a chair with shoes off and both feet flat on the ground. Rub your palms together and bring them into your heart center in a prayer position. Begin your ritual by tuning in with the "Adi Mantra"—"Ong Namo Guroo Dayv Namo"—three times.

Mantra

Play the "Kundalini Mantra for Self-Esteem and Confidence" as you warm up, and meditate. This mantra helps build up your self-esteem and confidence. We love the one by Bachan Kaur titled "Bountiful, Blissful, Beautiful."

With this mantra, you are declaring that at your core you are bountiful, bliss-ful, and beautiful. You know deep down that's who you are—your mind just needs to wrap itself around that fact.

Warm-Up

Sufi Grinds warm up your solar plexus—your energetic center for personal power, confidence, worthiness, and action.

Sitting in Easy Pose (or in a chair with your feet on the ground), place your hands on your knees and begin rotating the spine in a circular grinding motion. Lean to the right, make your way forward, to the left, and then circle back, rounding out your back. Your shoulders will remain over your hips, so it's not a huge or exagger-ated movement. It will warm up the spine, help with digestion, promote emotional stability, and build strength in your solar plexus.

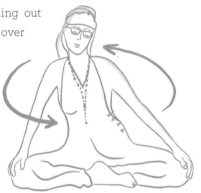

Complete twenty-six rotations, or one to two minutes, in each direction.

Inhale to center, hold the breath, and exhale out completely to relax.

Meditation

This meditation is called Experiencing the Original You.[15] It will help you develop personal excellence and give you a new concept of who you are.

PART 1

Posture. Sit in Easy Pose (a cross-legged position).

Mudra. Interlace your fingers and turn your hands so that the palms face outward. This is called Reverse Elbow Lock. Extend your arms straight out in front of you with no bend in the elbows. Stay steady and do not raise or lower your arms once you are in position.

Eyes. The eyes are focused at the tip of the nose.

Breath. Try to breathe only one breath per minute. Inhale for twenty seconds, hold for twenty seconds, and exhale for twenty seconds. Continue this long, slow, deep breath for three minutes. If you have problems with your stomach and digestion, your elbows may hurt or be uncomfortable in this exercise. If twenty seconds is difficult, start with equal increments of time—for instance, inhale for five seconds, hold for five, exhale for five. Work up to twenty seconds.

PART 2

Remain in position with the eyes focused at the tip of the nose. Continuously inhale through the nose and exhale through the mouth with the force of cannon fire. Continue for three minutes. How much you can heal yourself now will be in direct proportion to the strength of your breath.

PART 3

Remain in position. Inhale, hold your breath, and pump your navel. When you can no longer hold your breath, exhale. Immediately inhale and again pump your navel. Continue at your own breath rhythm, pumping your navel as vigorously as you can. Continue for three minutes.

To end. Inhale, hold the breath for fifteen seconds, and stretch your arms out as far as possible, putting pressure on your joined fingers. Exhale through the mouth like cannon fire. Repeat this sequence two more times.

To fully circulate the energy you have created, extend your Jupiter (pointer) fingers straight up and lock down the other three fingers with your thumb. Circle your forearms in outward circles as fast as possible. This movement has to be so vigorous that the entire spine moves. Continue for two and a half minutes. Inhale and relax your hands down.

Seal your practice with Sat Naam. Bring your hands together in Prayer Pose in front of your heart. Inhale deeply and either chant or say out loud "Sat Naam," which means "truth is my essence."

Journal

Write a love letter to yourself every morning for the forty days you commit to this ritual. Ask yourself what makes you unique and what you love about yourself. Watch what your mind does here—can you keep your comments positive?

The format is up to you—it can be an actual letter to yourself or you can write in list form. (We'd suggest up to ten things on the list each day.)

Save all the letters that you write for forty days and watch the progression from day one to forty. It will be fun on day forty to look back to day one to see how your letters to yourself have changed, shifted, and grown.

Affirmation

Begin repeating this affirmation in your mind:

My uniqueness is my gift to the world, and by showing up as me, I heal myself and everyone around me.

Visualization

Picture your most confident and worthy future self. Who are you? What do you look like? Where are you? Who are you talking to? What are you saying? What kind of energy are you carrying? Let your mind get lost with this and see yourself so clearly that it almost feels real. Stay here for three to five minutes before coming back to your breath. Inhale deeply, hold your breath, then exhale and relax.

Nourishment

Make yourself mint tea (we love 100 percent mint tea) to sip on while you get ready for your day. Mint is a plant that helps us feel better about ourselves because it brings joyful, light, bright, and fun energy to our bodies and our minds.

NICE WORK, BABE! YOU'RE BEAMING WITH CONFIDENCE AND LOVE FOR YOURSELF, AND YOU'RE ON A JOURNEY TO FINDING THE HIDDEN TREASURES BURIED WITHIN YOUR SOUL. THEY HAVE BEEN WAITING FOR YOU!

—XO, B+T

Radiant Being
Amplify Beauty and Your Aura

30-80 MINUTES

This ritual is all about amplifying your true inner beauty, which then shows up outwardly. Have you ever changed your opinion about how someone looked after getting to know them? They become more beautiful and radiant, and you're not sure why? That's what this ritual does. It's about projecting and expanding your aura and deciding how you want to show up in the world.

Why do we care about this aura thing? Because it's our greatest projector (energy to call in what we want) and protector (repels energy that isn't a match). It's an oval of light, the energy field around you. It's your vibration in motion and is essentially a culmination of your chakras and what you think, feel, and say. If the energy encompassing you is weak, you will feel trapped by negativity—it can make you physically ill, mentally insane, and spiritually inept. Your own vibration feeds your aura, and the weaker it is, the weaker the energy you're attracting.

The good news—actually, great news!—is that the opposite is true too. The stronger your energy field, the more magnetic you will be. When you are clear and connected mentally and are operating from a beautiful mind, it draws people to you and makes them feel amazing, regardless of the outfit you are wearing or whether you've had a moon-cycle breakout. All people will see is your glow.

This ritual is an overall energetic upgrade that will raise your vibration and balance out your whole system. On the other side of this commitment is living your best life, radiant skin, bright white eyes, and energy that lights up the room. Put on your crown: queen energy is coming through.

Gather

- Yoga mat, meditation cushion, or chair.

- Moonstone crystal. Place this in front of your mat for your meditation or wear a moonstone necklace during these forty days and beyond. It will help cleanse your aura and harmonize discordant vibrations, allowing you to tap into the calm, neutral, and elegant radiant-being vibes.

- Rose hip oil. After your self-care practice, mix a few drops of rose hip oil with almond oil, rub it together on your hands, and deeply breathe in its scent. Finish by massaging the oil onto your face or arms to moisturize and improve the appearance of age spots and wrinkles.

- Journal and pen.

- Ingredients for Alkaline Lime Water and a light breakfast of your choice.

Self-Care

Begin this ritual by heading over to your bathroom (or the loo, as the royals call it!) and splash cold water on your face in the sink. It's a form of hydrotherapy and wakes up your cells. Then head to your mat, beauty!

Warm-Up

Begin in a standing position to really get down and dirty and cleanse out that aura! This posture not only helps you set your protective shield for the day, but it also opens the heart chakra, gets your blood flowing, and rejuvenates your cells. Warning: You may feel tingly, but don't worry. It's just all that energy moving and shaking!

To begin, bring your feet shoulder-width distance apart, close your eyes, and focus at your third-eye chakra (between the eyebrows). Inhale deeply and sweep your arms out by the sides of your body and up until your palms meet briefly overhead. Exhale powerfully and sweep the arms back down to the sides of the legs, as if they were wings of a great bird or a paintbrush. Continue this motion and breath for at least three minutes. Then, slowly come to sitting silently and still for one minute to feel the aura and its vastness.

Journal

Sit quietly and ask the question, "Who am I? What is my truth? Where does my beauty lie? What are my greatest gifts?" Then just listen...silently. And then listen more. And more.

Write down what you hear, even if it's just a few bullet points.

Tune In

Still sitting in a cross-legged position, or alternatively, you can sit in a chair with shoes off and both feet flat on the ground, rub your palms together and bring them into your heart center in a prayer position. Begin your ritual by tuning in with the "Adi Mantra"—"Ong Namo Guroo Dayv Namo"—three times.

Mantra

For the breathwork and warm-up portions of the ritual, play the mantra "Bliss (I Am the Light of My Soul)" by Sirgun Kaur and Sat Darshan Singh. It will penetrate the subconscious with this truth: *I am the light of the soul. I am bountiful. I am beautiful. I am bliss. I am, I am.* (You can find it on the Spotify playlist we made to accompany this book!)

Breathwork

Now we are going to go into the equivalent of a dry-brush and salt-scrub sesh for your aura: *Sitali Pranayam*. We call this the glow breath, because it's extremely beautifying—our Kundalini version of face yoga. (That's a thing, if you haven't heard!)

Sit in a comfortable, meditative posture with a straight spine. Curl the tongue up on the sides and protrude it slightly past the lips. Inhale deeply and smoothly through the rolled tongue, expanding your stomach out, and then close your mouth and exhale through the nose, contracting the abdomen in toward your spine. Continue twenty-six times—it should take you around two to two and a half minutes.

To finish, inhale, hold the breath, pull the tongue in, and relax. If your tongue tastes bitter at first, it's a sign that toxins are present in your body. But as you continue through the forty days, your tongue will taste sweeter—a sign that you are detoxing that aura and any low vibes inside!

End your day with twenty-six more of these bad boys...glowy babe alert!

Affirmation

To really drive this home, repeat the mantra you have been listening to and make it your affirmation. Say it five times, either to yourself or out loud, and feel into this truth:

> *I am the light of the soul. I am bountiful. I am beautiful. I am bliss. I am, I am.*

Meditation

For this ritual's meditation, we're tapping into the compassion of the universe to expand and uplift us. This creates a divine shield from the universe to accompany you—kind of like your own personal energetic Wonder Woman cape.

The following meditation blows the doors off of your beauty and extends the aura so its outer arc acts as a filter and a connector to the universal magnetic field, helping you become more positive, more fearless and happier. Nothing will get in your way!

Posture + Mudra. Sit down with your legs out in front of you. Bring your right knee in close to your chest with your right foot flat on the ground, toes pointing straight ahead. Place the sole of your left foot against the arch and ankle of your right foot. The ball of your left foot rests just in front of the ankle bone of your right foot.

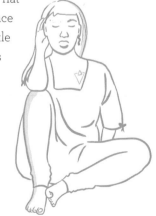

Make a fist with your left hand and place it on the ground beside your left hip. Use this to balance the posture. Bend your right elbow and place it on top of your right knee. Bring your right hand back along the side of your head with the palm facing your ear. Form a shallow cup of the right palm. Then bring it against the skull so it contacts the skull below the ear but stays open above the ear. It is as if you formed a cup of the hand to amplify a faint sound that you want to hear.

Eyes. Eyes are closed and focused at the brow point.

Mantra. Inhale deeply and chant "Maaa" in a long, full, smooth sound. Project the sound as if someone were listening to you. As you chant, listen to the sound and let it vibrate through your whole body. If you chant in a group, hear the overtones that develop and let those tones vibrate all around you and in every cell of your body.

In this meditation, the sound of "Maaa" opens the heart center and expands your aura, increases your radiance, and calls on compassion and protection. It is the sound that a baby uses to call on the mother. Here, your soul is the child, and the universe becomes the mother. If you call, she will come to your aid and comfort.

Chant the mantra at a comfortable, high pitch. When you have exhaled completely, take another deep breath and continue.

Time. Continue for eleven to thirty-one minutes.

Switch sides. Then change the legs and hands to the other side. Continue for an equal amount of time. Start slowly. Learn to hold the concentration into the sound.

If you want to, you can build the meditation on each side to total sixty-two minutes...ascension vibes to the max!

To end. Feel free to come onto your back for a one- to three-minute relaxation, letting all of this beautiful energy settle and recalibrate in your system.

Seal your practice with Sat Naam: Bring your hands together in Prayer Pose in front of your heart. Inhale deeply and either chant or say out loud "Sat Naam," which means "truth is my essence."

Nourishment

If you crave comfort foods and tend to overeat, it's a sign that your aura is weak. A lot of times we can look to heavy foods to make us feel secure, or we desire things like soda or coffee to experience a fake sense of expansion. But really, these are all just things that your soul is craving through the strengthening of your aura.

At the end of this ritual, eat a light breakfast, like cut-up bananas or berries to help your mind and body flush and restore. If you need more substance, drizzle almond butter over them.

Then, end with a glass of Alkaline Lime Water. To make, squeeze a full lime (Key lime, if possible) into a full glass of spring water. This drink provides many benefits, like improved digestion, balanced pH, clearer skin, and other radiant-being results you deserve.

If you feel food cravings kicking in, do jumping jacks or Ego Eradicator (found in ritual 4, "The Gold Rush") or take a cold shower to shift the energy. You can also seek help from Archangel Raphael, the angel of healing. All you have to do is pray or meditate to Raphael and ask him to help you transform your diet in a way that enhances your beauty and expands your aura.[16]

> **REMEMBER, YOU ARE A RADIANT BEING OF LIGHT WHO CAME HERE TO PLANET EARTH AS A SPIRITUAL BEING IN A HUMAN BODY.** IT'S WHO YOU ARE. IT'S JUST ABOUT REMEMBERING AGAIN AND AGAIN, AND WE'RE HERE FOR YOU IF YOU EVER FORGET.
>
> *—XO, B+T*

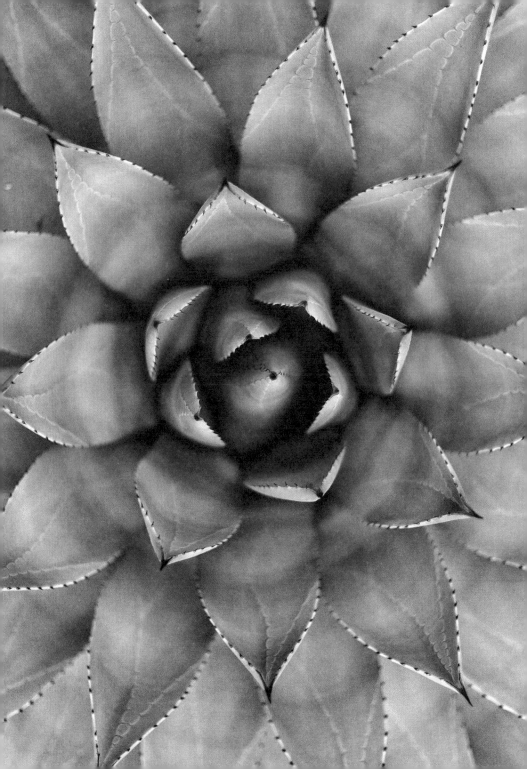

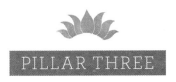

Connecting to You

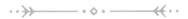

We've all heard that new-age phrase "Be your own guru," right? Well, this is a "new-age" phrase for a reason—because, until very recently, we humans have been experiencing the astrological Age of Pisces—a time in which society was dominated by social hierarchy, power, and structured religion. No one was their own guru. We were told what to believe and to look outside of ourselves for something or someone to help us connect to the Divine, activate our voices, and discover our destiny. For the last two thousand years, this is the energy within which our ancestors have been operating. But all that has changed.

Around November 11, 2011, we said sayonara to the Age of Pisces and moved into the new Age of Aquarius. (Astrologers have varying opinions on the exact date of the transition.) Suddenly, being your own guru became the cool thing to do.

The Aquarian Age is sometimes called the "Information Age" or the "Age of Experience" because we now have access to all the resources and knowledge disseminated by our BFF: the internet. Information used to be largely contained within a select group of elite people—teachers, religious leaders, and gurus. If you didn't know something or wanted to make sense of your experience, you had to rely on others to show you the way based on their beliefs. Now, thanks to our mobile phones, computers, and tablets, all the information in the world is readily available to everyone. If you want to chart a new path for yourself, you can get instant inspiration by entering a few words into a search engine. Ancient and sacred knowledge, rituals from cultures all around the world, scientific studies, astronomy, ancient astrology, history, current news (real and fake)—you can now immerse yourself in whatever knowledge you want, figure out what feels true for you, and put it into practice. You decide you want to learn about the ancient Egyptians. Pull up Amazon.com or Audible and find yourself one of the hundreds of books available, and in two minutes with a few clicks of a button, you're ready to begin learning everything about this civilization. It's actually kind of crazy to think about how easy it is.

With all this knowledge at your fingertips, you don't need to depend as much on other people to shape your worldview. You get to be your own guru. This makes it easier to tap into your intuition, activate your voice, and discover your destiny on your own terms, and in your own timing. Seriously, what an amazing time to live—it's so empowering!

It's now your own personal responsibility to develop this connection to your inner self. When you do this, you win at life. You develop unwavering confidence. You speak your truth to those you hold close and to the masses. You follow your gut and don't have to work as hard trying to make things happen because you're guided to your best life every day. Your life is happening with you and for you. Most of all, when you develop a strong connection to yourself, you can align with your gifts and activate your destiny.

We created the rituals in this section so you can experience your own personal victory and feel the deep satisfaction that comes with having a strong connection to you and all that you are, because at the core of you is a perfect, ecstatic, radiant being who does not waiver from being and emanating love.

If you're not familiar with the astrological ages, here's a quick explanation: The Earth rotates on an axis with a slight circular wobble to it, like a spinning top. This is called axial precision. Every twenty-six thousand years or so, that wobble completes a full circle. This circle is divided into twelve parts represented by the twelve zodiac signs (around twenty-one hundred years for each sign). When the shift between ages happens, big changes come along with it.[17]

RITUAL 8 >>>

Connect to the Divine
Intuitive Activation

15–25 MINUTES

We like to think of intuition as our ever-present GPS system…more like Waze, to be exact. If you're not familiar with the app, it very accurately tracks traffic jams, accidents, and anything that changes on your route so you can plan your journey most efficiently. In a similar way, your intuition is that little voice in your ear that steers you toward the people, places, and situations that will best serve you, and alerts you when you need to change course. As you develop this gift, even if you don't quite understand why you're being guided down a certain path, you begin to trust it, follow it, and know that it will take you in the direction of your highest good.

You don't have to be a fourteenth-generation medium or spiritual guru to tap into this gift—although you can be, of course! Every single person can activate their intuition and, unlike other forms of expert guidance, it's free.

The thing is, many people are more connected to their Instagram feeds or the news headlines than their own intuition. This brings confusion, loneliness, and fear, all major side effects of flying blind without your inner GPS—that connection to intelligence that is more intelligent than you!

But what *is* intuition? Although it's largely an intangible concept, it is physically connected to a specific place in our bodies: the pineal gland, or sixth chakra (aka the *ajna*, or third-eye, chakra). Philosopher René Descartes referred to the pineal gland—which produces melatonin and affects our sleep cycles—as the "principal seat of the soul," where the body and spirit meet.[18] From a yogic perspective, the sixth chakra allows us to see the unseen and operate from a deep inner knowing. The pineal gland can be negatively affected by a number of proven factors, including calcium buildup, fluoride and other chemicals in water, pesticides and herbicides, and heavy metals.[19] An imbalanced pineal gland is linked with all sorts of things that totally mess with our high vibes, like insomnia, depression, hormone imbalances, and Alzheimer's disease.[20] For us, this was some major motivation to prioritize our pineal gland health and supercharge our intuition...anyone else?

If you invest a little bit of time each day to strengthen your intuition, you end up getting *so* much in return. You save energy you once spent worrying about the future. You save time you once wasted trying to figure things out alone. And you gain a strong knowing that your challenges are here to make you stronger. You start to truly trust that you are learning the best lesson to take you to better places, versus thinking, *Whyyyy me, universe? I hate you, nothing is working! I give up and accept my calcified pineal gland and mediocre life.*

Basically, you become like a cheetah: unstoppable not because of the speed at which you move through life, but because of your ability to see clearly and to change directions quickly.[21] That is what intuition gives us, and that is what we will do in this ritual.

Gather

- Yoga mat, meditation cushion, or chair.

- Clear quartz crystal. This crystal promotes clarity of mind and allows you to hear any messages that want to come through. Hold it in one hand during the breathwork portion of this ritual.

- Almond or coconut oil. You'll use it for a little self-massage during the first part of this ritual!

- Ingredients for the Third-Eye-Boosting Breakfast.

Tune In

Come down onto your mat, sitting in a cross-legged position. Alternatively, you can sit in a chair with shoes off and both feet flat on the ground. Rub your palms together and bring them into your heart center in a prayer position. Begin your ritual by tuning in with the "Adi Mantra"—"Ong Namo Guroo Dayv Namo"—three times.

Breathwork + Self-Care + Mantra

Close your eyes while turning your gaze inward and up to connect to your third eye—the point between your eyebrows. Breathe long and deep three times, creating a cosmic connection and becoming aware of this divine gateway to your inner guidance system. Now, to activate it even more, gently massage your third eye with almond or coconut oil in clockwise circles for fifteen to thirty seconds.

Continue to breathe long and deep as your turn on the "Wah Yantee" mantra and listen to it for three minutes. (We love Nirinjan Kaur Khalsa's version!) This mantra awakens your intuition and has been chanted for over two thousand years, which charges it with blessings. You can opt to chant along to really activate it into your aura.

Wah Yantee, Kaar Yantee,

Jagat Utpatee, Aadak It Whaa-haa

Brahmaaday Trayshaa Guroo

It Whaa-hay Guroo.

This mantra calls the higher self—the creative self—to come through from the purest source energy. It's about moving from the darkness so you can see and be the light.

Warm-Up

Get ready to sweat! This exercise will help rebalance your magnetic field and strengthen your nervous system in preparation for the meditation that follows.[22]

Stand up straight. Put the right foot slightly forward. Stretch the left leg far backward. Place the top of the left foot on the ground. Extend the arms forward parallel to the ground. Bring the palms together. Tilt the spine slightly forward of the vertical position. Fix the eyes on the horizon or at the brow point.

Take a deep breath, then begin a rhythmic chant of "Sat Naam." Emphasize the sound "Sat" as you pull the navel point (the energy center located two to three inches below the belly button) in and lightly squeeze your pelvic floor. Continue for one and a half minutes. (You can slowly build up to seven and a half minutes over time.) Then inhale. Relax.

Switch and place the left leg forward. Repeat the exercise for an equal period of time.

Meditation

Now feel free to shake out your legs and grab a sip of water before we get into the Activate Your Intuition Meditation.[23] This technology tunes up our intuition muscle, heightening our abilities and allowing us to trust them.

Posture. Sit in a comfortable seated position.

Mudra. Place the hands together in Prayer Pose. Keep the Jupiter (index) fingers extended as you interlock the other fingers to clasp the two hands together. Cross the thumbs. (It'll look like a Charlie's Angels handgun.) Place the mudra a little below your nose where you can look at the tips of the Jupiter fingers through a one-tenth opening of your eyes.

Eyes. Eyes are one-tenth open.

Breath. Make an O shape with the mouth and inhale in four powerful, four-second breaths through the mouth. Exhale in one powerful, one-second breath through the nose. Be sure to really inhale heavily through the mouth and push the breath out through the nose—you are using your own breath and diaphragm to move your energy and open the chakras, and the more strongly you do this, the greater the results.

Time. Continue this breath pattern for sixteen minutes.

To end. Sit up straight. Inhale, hold the breath for twenty seconds, and stretch the arms out to the sides, palms facing upward. This will give you power to balance the central spinal column. Exhale. Inhale deep, hold the breath for twenty seconds, stretch the arms horizontally, and stretch the spine vertically. Make a T square. Exhale. Inhale deep, hold the breath for twenty seconds, and open up the fingers, making them like steel. Squeeze your entire energy and bring it into your arms. Exhale and relax.

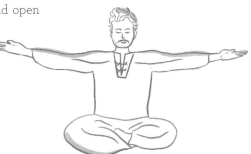

Seal your practice with Sat Naam. Bring your hands together in Prayer Pose in front of your heart. Inhale deeply and either chant or say out loud "Sat Naam," which means "truth is my essence."

Affirmation

After the meditation, sit in silence and repeat the following affirmation three to five times to yourself or out loud.

> *I am connected and guided. I trust my intuitive abilities to direct me on my highest path and provide me with everything I need.*

If any doubts come up, they are leaving your subconscious—simply say, "I release you." Feel the energy of this affirmation as you repeat it three to five times to yourself or out loud. You can even choose to write it down three to five times and journal about what it feels like for this to be true.

Visualization

Now take a minute and visualize yourself going throughout your day with the voice of your inner GPS system in your ear. How does it make you feel? How does it change your confidence and your choices? Feel that liberation and see what it looks like for you, you hot cheetah!

Nourishment

Now that you're feeling fierce, it's time to up your nutrition to support all the amazing work you just did. This part of the ritual is super simple, but it includes ingredients that are linked to a strong intuition. Both lime and blueberries are rich in antioxidants and vitamin C, which help the liver flush toxins from your body that may sabotage the pineal gland.

THIRD-EYE-BOOSTING BREAKFAST

Prep time: 2 minutes
Makes 1 serving

1 cup spring or alkaline water (not tap water)

¼ lime, preferably Key lime

1 handful of blueberries

>> Warm the water to a lukewarm temperature. Squeeze ¼ lime into the water and save the rest for tomorrow. Eat the handful of blueberries or add them to your favorite oatmeal or smoothie. Enjoy the intuition-enhancing effects of these simple nourishment practices!

To take intuitive nutrition to the next level, you can go on a decalcification program—aka a clairvoyant diet! It involves cutting out meat, dairy, alcohol, caffeine, sugar, tobacco, and large fish (or eating less of these things) while drinking two liters of alkaline or spring water daily. Eat lots of green foods and rainbow-colored whole foods, like grapes, cabbage, oranges, pears, bananas, kale, and pumpkin. Here are some other great foods to add to your diet: chlorella, cacao, garlic, lemons, apple cider vinegar, beets, oregano oil, raw foods, and superfoods like shilajit, goji berries, coconut oil, and maca powder. Also, use nontoxic makeup and products as much as possible. Check out our free nontoxic guide on our website!

❝❞

TRUST THAT YOU HAVE EVERYTHING YOU NEED INSIDE OF YOU! YOU HAVE THE ABILITY TO TAP INTO YOUR INNER KNOWING AND RECEIVE ALL THE ANSWERS YOU NEED. CONTINUE TO DEVELOP AND STRENGTHEN THIS CONNECTION—IT'S A JOURNEY, BUT YOU'RE ALREADY ON YOUR WAY!

—XO, B+T

Activate Your Voice
Be Seen and Heard

20 MINUTES

You don't have to be a Grammy-winning singer or an activist who protests on the side of the road to have a powerful voice that influences people and creates change. But for lots of people, the thought of open self-expression is straight-up scary.

There are so many different reasons that keep people from using their voice to express their wants, needs, desires, and perceptions. We all have a powerful message inside us, but we give ourselves permission to dim our light and hide behind a shield of protection because of past experiences and the stories we hold on to. So what's keeping you from standing tall, taking a stand for what you believe, and sharing it with the world?

Maybe some of these thoughts sound familiar: *People don't like the way my voice sounds. I won't be accepted or taken seriously if I share the real me. Saying how I feel is not a battle worth fighting. What if they think I'm stupid or I can't explain myself clearly?* This kind of inner dialogue keeps you suppressed and struggling to manifest the life you have been dreaming of. But none of these stories is true. Believe it or not, it's your birthright to express all of who you are without fear of being judged, rejected, or belittled. You deserve to be seen and heard for the simple fact that you are you.

Not only that, but your words also cast spells that create your reality—they are the seeds planted for your manifestations to come. (Think about the word "spelling"!) Your voice is your human superpower, your magic wand in this physical world. It's time to start having fun with it!

Whether you're an aspiring motivational speaker or someone who wants to nail that big presentation at work, someone who wants to have better communication with loved ones or someone who wants to fall in love with their own voice—this ritual was created for you. It will activate your voice current, open up your throat chakra (aka your communication command center), and give you the power of projection to command attention in any room. Your voice will become your superpower.

Are you ready to activate that voice, love? Let's go!

"

GROWING UP, SHARING HOW I FELT WASN'T ALWAYS RECEIVED WELL. I LEARNED IT WAS BEST TO SUPPRESS MY EMOTIONS AND MY THOUGHTS IF THEY WERE GOING TO RUFFLE TOO MANY FEATHERS. I LEARNED THAT IF I WENT WITH THE FLOW, PEOPLE WOULD LIKE ME, AND I'D HAVE MORE FRIENDS. I LEARNED TO EXCEL IN LIFE BY KEEPING QUIET. I CLOSED MYSELF OFF, AND THEN I WONDERED WHY PEOPLE WOULD OFTEN NOT REMEMBER MEETING ME, BUT THEY'D REMEMBER THE FRIEND I WAS WITH. I FELT FORGETTABLE AND GOT REALLY GOOD AT BEING UNSEEN. FOR A WHILE I FORGOT HOW TO BE ANYONE ELSE. I GOT FED UP WITH THIS OLD STORY, WENT DEEPER INWARD, AND REALIZED I HAD THIS SHIELD UP BECAUSE I THOUGHT IT WOULD PROTECT ME. BUT ALL IT DID WAS KEEP ME FROM EVERYTHING I WANTED. **IT KEPT ME HIDDEN FROM THE WORLD AND DISTRACTED ME FROM REALLY GETTING TO KNOW MYSELF BECAUSE I WAS ALWAYS LOOKING FOR SOMEONE TO SEE ME AND SAVE ME.** I BEGAN TO CONNECT TO WHO I WAS, ACTIVATE MY VOICE, AND ALLOW MYSELF TO BE SEEN WITH THIS RITUAL, AND IT HAS GIVEN ME ABSOLUTE FREEDOM OF EXPRESSION THAT'S EXPANDING EVERY DAY.

—Tara

Gather

- Yoga mat, meditation cushion, or chair.

- Azurite crystal. Azurite vibrates with the higher energy centers, helps remove blocks in the throat chakra, and develops psychic communication gifts. Meditate with this crystal through the ritual, and if you're feeling called to, wear it as a necklace to help activate the throat chakra.

- Nasya oil. We love to use this Ayurvedic oil to soothe seasonal allergies, lubricate our nasal passages, and keep our throats feeling healthy. (Especially in the winter!) After you complete this ritual, tilt your head back, place a few drops in each nostril, and sniff so you feel the oil coating your throat.

- Ingredients for Ginger Aloe Vera Tea.

Tune In

Come down onto your mat, sitting in a cross-legged position. Alternatively, you can sit in a chair with shoes off and both feet flat on the ground. Rub your palms together and bring them into your heart center in a prayer position. Begin your ritual by tuning in with the "Adi Mantra"—"Ong Namo Guroo Dayv Namo"—three times.

Mantra

We'll use the "Humee Hum Brahm Hum" mantra for the entire ritual—it translates to "We are we, we are God." You'll play it during the warm-up, breathwork, and meditation portions.

Chanting "Humee Hum Brahm Hum" connects you to the spirit of the universe and allows it to flow through you via your voice. (Remember the scene in

The Little Mermaid where Ariel gets her voice back? This mantra does the same thing.)

We love Nirinjan Kaur's version titled "Humee Hum" from the album *Musical Affirmations Collection Volume 2*. You can find it on the Spotify playlist that we made for this book!

Breathwork

We'll start activating our voices with a powerful Kundalini breathwork practice called Lion's Breath. It will clear the upper chest and throat of stagnant energy that has been keeping you from letting your voice shine. Plus, it is said to help cleanse toxins in this area, pushing them into the lymphatic system, and it's good for the health of your thyroid. Win, win, win!

You can practice this breathwork in a cross-legged position, sitting on your heels, or in a chair with your feet on the ground. Sit up tall and place your hands on your knees. Extend your tongue out to touch the chin—you'll look like a lion panting. Keeping your tongue out, begin to breathe powerfully, forcing the breath over the tongue, without any rasping. As you inhale, expand the stomach out. On the exhale, contract the stomach in. Close your eyes. Keep a steady pace with powerful breaths, slowly increasing your speed.

Continue for two minutes.

To end, inhale with the tongue out and hold the breath for five to ten seconds. Then exhale all the breath out completely.

Warm-Up

Sitting in the same position, place your hands on your knees. Inhale through the nose, shrugging your shoulders up to your ears, exhale, and release them down. Breathe from your belly and be sure to keep your arms relaxed and your eyes closed. Once you get going in a good rhythm, speed up the movement to a rapid pace.

Continue for one minute.

To end, deeply inhale, shrug your shoulders up toward your ears, and hold the breath for five to ten seconds. Exhale and release the shoulders down.

Meditation

To activate your voice, you have to exercise it. So, no surprise, during this meditation, you'll be using your voice to chant a now-familiar mantra—"Humee Hum Brahm Hum"—for eleven minutes.

This meditation can give you the power to create effective communication.[24] This doesn't just mean being able to speak clearly or hold another's attention, but also the ability to listen to what others are saying. It will activate your voice, balance your throat chakra, and relax the muscles in your neck so your voice can effortlessly flow through you.

Posture. Sit in Easy Pose with a straight spine. Create a firm Neck Lock by pulling your chin down and back so your neck is in line with the rest of your spine.

Mudra. The arms are straight, and the hands are in Gyan Mudra (thumbs and index fingertips touching) resting on the knees, palms facing up.

Eyes. Focus at the tip of the nose with eyes open. If this is too advanced, work up to it by closing your eyes and directing your eye gaze toward the tip of your nose.

Mantra. Chant the "Humee Hum" mantra with the root of the tongue. Keep that firm Neck Lock in place.

Time. Continue to chant for eleven minutes, working up to twenty-two minutes per practice over time.

Seal your practice with Sat Naam. Bring your hands together in Prayer Pose in front of your heart. Inhale deeply and either chant or say out loud "Sat Naam," which means "truth is my essence."

Visualization + Affirmation

Sit in silence after you've completed the meditation and feel the pulsating energy coming from your throat. Keep your focus on this area of your body and visualize a bright blue ball of light spinning counterclockwise, getting brighter and brighter with every revolution. Then, move your attention outward to the energy field around your body—your aura—and pulsate this blue light into your energy field.

Now, imagine yourself dropping the shield around you that keeps people from seeing this bright radiant energy you're creating. Imagine yourself standing in front of someone or a group of people who are eager to hear your message. They cannot wait to hear you speak. Bask in that feeling. Now visualize your voice coming out eloquently and fearlessly, and repeat the affirmation:

I am safe to express myself with clarity and confidence.

Nourishment

Head to the kitchen to seal the ritual with a simple, but powerful, voice-supporting Ginger Aloe Vera Tea. Ginger helps alleviate symptoms of respiratory ailments including, asthma, coughs, and bronchitis—all things that affect our voices—and the aloe helps to reduce inflammation to support a healthy throat.

GINGER ALOE VERA TEA

Prep time: 20 minutes
Makes 2 servings

2 cups filtered water

4–5 slices fresh ginger, peeled (Slice the ginger ahead of time to cut down on prep time. You can also use ginger tea bags.)

1 teaspoon aloe vera gel (For the freshest gel, scoop out the jelly from an aloe vera plant leaf, or you can buy it packaged.)

Maple syrup to taste

>> Bring the water and ginger slices to a boil, then reduce heat and simmer uncovered for ten to fifteen minutes until the water is dark and smells strongly of ginger. Strain the ginger water into a mug and scoop the aloe vera gel into the tea. Add maple syrup to taste. Enjoy!

ALLOW YOURSELF TO RELAX AS YOU SPEAK TODAY. LET THE ENERGY OF THE MANTRA "HUMEE HUM BRAHM HUM" COME THROUGH YOUR VOICE IN EVERY INTERACTION. **SLOW YOUR SPEECH, SPEAK FROM THE HEART, DROP YOUR SHIELD AND LET YOURSELF BE SEEN,** AND SET THE INTENTION TO ACTIVELY LISTEN TO OTHERS TODAY. HAVE AN AMAZING DAY, BABE— GET OUT THERE AND USE YOUR SUPERPOWER!

—XO, B+T

RITUAL 10 >>>

Discover Your Destiny
Find and Fulfill Your Purpose

15-25 MINUTES

One of the most common questions we get asked is, "How do I find my purpose in life?" It's a great question to ask, but we think the idea of "finding" your reason for being is a little misleading. We have discovered that it's not about actively seeking for anything—it's about returning to yourself so your purpose is illuminated within *you*.

The first step in this process is to start cleansing away everything that is not you and doesn't connect back to your "why." Through opening our chakras with Kundalini yoga, we are able to increase our consciousness and see our truth clearly. This allows us to become aware of our highest destiny and attract it to us. You may also realize that you need to let go of a life you thought you should be living, identities that you have held on to tightly, or people who aren't a match anymore. But on the other side of that is the life you truly want and were born to live. When you align with your purpose, the universe conspires in your favor and helps you in some of the most unexpected ways.

That is how it has been for us on this journey. After we started working with our Kundalini energy, we both left our corporate careers and our old identities and stepped completely outside of our comfort zones. We balanced our chakras and released so much energy that was not true to our individual souls, which then increased our consciousness and awareness. At the time, we were closer to our inner selves than we'd ever been, and it felt amazing. We could feel something big was trying to reveal itself, but we needed to align with it…and we did. We were able to receive a remarkably vivid vision of working together on this mission to elevate consciousness on the planet.

Although it's not always unicorns and rainbows and it takes courage and strength, on the other side are big rewards. This ritual will help you elevate your consciousness so you can get clear on who you really are and pursue your purpose fearlessly. When you do this, you inspire others to do the same just by being you, and that is how we can all elevate the globe.

The only question is, are you ready for the journey?

66 99

WHEN MY MOM, AT AGE FIFTY-FIVE, PASSED AWAY IN MY ARMS, I STARTED TO CARE MORE THAN EVER ABOUT WHY I'M ON THIS PLANET AND WHAT I'M HERE TO DO. I FELT A SENSE OF URGENCY TO GET IT DONE AND HAVE A DAMN GOOD TIME DOING IT. ALTHOUGH I HAD HEARD MESSAGES A MILLION TIMES, LIKE, 'LIVE LIKE YOU'LL DIE TOMORROW,' AND 'IN THE END, YOU'LL ONLY REGRET THE CHANCES YOU DIDN'T TAKE,' IT WASN'T UNTIL THAT MOMENT THAT I ACTUALLY GOT THEM. I UNDERSTOOD THAT I WASN'T LIVING IN ALIGNMENT WITH MY TRUTH YET, AND I KNEW THAT WAS GOING TO BE MY NUMBER-ONE PRIORITY MOVING FORWARD. NOTHING ELSE REALLY MATTERS. THAT IS WHAT GOT ME GOING BIG TIME, AND IT'S THE WHY THAT CONTINUES TO DRIVE ME TO LIVE IN ACCORDANCE WITH MY PURPOSE AND VALUES.

—Britt

Gather

- Yoga mat, meditation cushion, or chair.

- Lapis lazuli crystal. Lapis lazuli will help you to pursue your true destiny and connect you to your inner wisdom. You can wear this stone as a piece of jewelry to help you stay on track.

- Ingredients for the Vegan Golden Milk Latte.

Tune In

Come down onto your mat, sitting in a cross-legged position. Alternatively, you can sit in a chair with shoes off and both feet flat on the ground. Rub your palms together and bring them into your heart center in a prayer position. Begin your ritual by tuning in with the "Adi Mantra"—"Ong Namo Guroo Dayv Namo"—three times.

Mantra

Begin to play the highest of all the mantras, the "Mul Mantra." This mantra contains the root sound that is the basis of all effective mantras and helps us to stay in a perfect flow with the universe. It's said that its vibration is so powerful that it can change your fate and help you rewrite your destiny. We love the "Mul Mantra (Extended Version)" single from White Sun. You can find it on the Spotify playlist we made for this book.

Ek Ong Kaar, Sat Naam, Kartaa Purakh, Nirbho, Nirvair

Akal Morrt, Ajoonee, Saibhang, Gurprasaad. Jap

Aad Such, Jugad Such, Haibhee Such

Naanak Hosee Bhee Such

Play the "Mul Mantra" throughout your day, sing along with it in the car, play it at your desk, or listen to it when you're working around the house to keep your compass pointing in the direction of your destiny.

Warm-Up

When we're discovering and becoming a vibrational match to our destiny, we often need to clear out the aura and generate more energy to charge up the mind and all the body systems. That's what we'll be doing in this portion of the ritual. We'd recommend wearing a head covering—like a scarf or beanie—to contain the energy that you'll be creating with this meditation.

Come up to a standing position with your feet hip-width distance apart (two to three feet apart) for Windmill. You also can sit in a chair for this and place your feet on either side of the chair.

Raise your arms out to your sides, parallel to the ground, palms facing the floor.

Inhale deeply, and as you exhale, bend forward from the waist and bring your left palm down to your right foot (or your ankle or shin). Inhale as you come back to center with both arms out. Exhale as you bend from the waist and bring your right palm down to your left foot, ankle, or shin. Inhale and come back to center, continuing to alternate sides.

Keep moving for three minutes.

To end, inhale deeply to center with arms parallel to the ground and hold the breath for five to ten seconds. Exhale and relax the arms down. Come into a seated position or sitting in a chair with both feet on the ground.

Meditation

Sit in Easy Pose (a cross-legged position). You can sit on your heels if that's more comfortable. Create a light Neck Lock by pulling your chin slightly down and back so you feel pressure at the back of your neck.

Mudra. Make both hands into Lion's Paws: curl and tighten the fingers of each hand like lion's paws. Keep the tension in the hands throughout the exercise. Extend both arms out to the sides, parallel to the ground with the palms up.

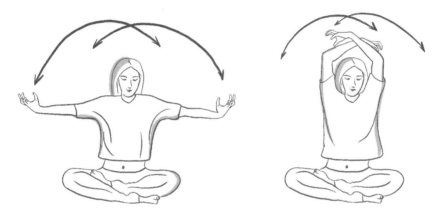

Movement. Bring both arms up over the head so the hands pass each other over the crown of the head. The elbows bend, and the palms face down. Then bring the hands back down as you extend the arms out parallel to the ground again. Start a rhythmic motion in this way. Alternate which wrist is in front when they cross each other over the head. The arm motion is very fast paced.

Breath. Inhale as the arms extend out and exhale as the arms cross over the head. As you increase the speed of the movement, the breath becomes a steady Breath of Fire where you inhale and exhale, equal in strength and length, through the nose. Allow the navel point (the energy center located two to three inches below the belly button) to move with the breath, expanding on the inhale, contracting on the exhale.[25] Note: If you're on the first three days of your moon cycle or you're pregnant, do long, deep breathing instead.

Time. Continue for nine minutes.

To end. Without breaking the pace of the exercise, stick the tongue out and down all the way. Continue for fifteen seconds more.

Then inhale, bring in the tongue, and fix the arms so that they form a sixty-degree arc around the head with the palms facing down about six inches apart over the head. The hands are still in Lion's Paws.

Hold the breath for fifteen seconds. Keep the arms fixed as you exhale and inhale completely through the nose. Then hold the breath for thirty seconds. Relax and let the arms down. Meditate at the heart center. Follow the gentle flow of the breath.

Begin to chant along with the "Mul Mantra" for three to five minutes.

Seal your practice with Sat Naam. Bring your hands together in Prayer Pose in front of your heart. Inhale deeply and either chant or say out loud "Sat Naam," which means "truth is my essence."

Affirmation

Before you get up from your meditation, say to yourself out loud:

I will show up 100 percent for everything in my path today.

Then, go out in the world and do just that. Show up 100 percent for the barista at the coffee shop and the woman who smiles at you walking down the street—be present in the moment and connect with them. You never know who has a message for you—who you will attract, or what opportunity may come your way today, but by showing up 100 percent for every moment, you will affirm to the universe that you are ready for it.

> 66 99
>
> THE AFFIRMATION IN THIS RITUAL IS THE SAME ONE I USED TO DISCOVER AND ALIGN WITH MY DESTINY. I BEGAN TO LIVE THIS AFFIRMATION, AND IT'S THE VERY REASON I RECEIVED THE VISION WITH BRITT TO START ELEVATE THE GLOBE. HAD I NOT SHOWN UP 100 PERCENT FOR THE OPPORTUNITY TO GO WITH HER TO SEE A HEALER IN NEW YORK—AFTER WHICH WE RECEIVED THE VISION FOR ELEVATE THE GLOBE TOGETHER—MY WHOLE STORY WOULD BE DIFFERENT. I'M SURE IT WOULD HAVE STILL BEEN GREAT BECAUSE I WAS ACTIVELY ON A PATH TO DISCOVER MY DESTINY, BUT THIS AFFIRMATION TOOK EVERYTHING TO ANOTHER LEVEL FOR ME.
>
> *—Tara*

Nourishment

After you've finished with your meditation and created all that new energy in your body, head over to the kitchen and make a Vegan Golden Milk Latte. The main ingredient is turmeric, which reduces inflammation and supports and soothes the nervous system you're strengthening. You're on your way to being able to handle anything thrown at you!

VEGAN GOLDEN MILK LATTE

Prep time: 10 minutes
Makes 1 serving

1 ½ cups almond milk

1 tablespoon coconut oil

1 teaspoon ground turmeric

1 teaspoon ground cinnamon

Pinch of black pepper and sea salt

1 tablespoon maple syrup (optional)

>> Mix the almond milk and coconut oil in a medium saucepan for five or six minutes or until warmed. Whisk in the rest of the ingredients. Stir until the mixture is frothy. Top with a sprinkle of cinnamon and serve.

SIP ON YOUR VEGAN GOLDEN MILK LATTE AT HOME OR TAKE IT TO GO. GET OUT THERE TODAY AND SHOW THE UNIVERSE THAT YOU'RE READY, YOUR DESTINY IS YOURS, AND YOU'RE SHOWING UP 100 PERCENT FOR EVERYTHING IN YOUR PATH TO GETTING THERE. WE ARE SO EXCITED FOR YOU!

—XO, B+T

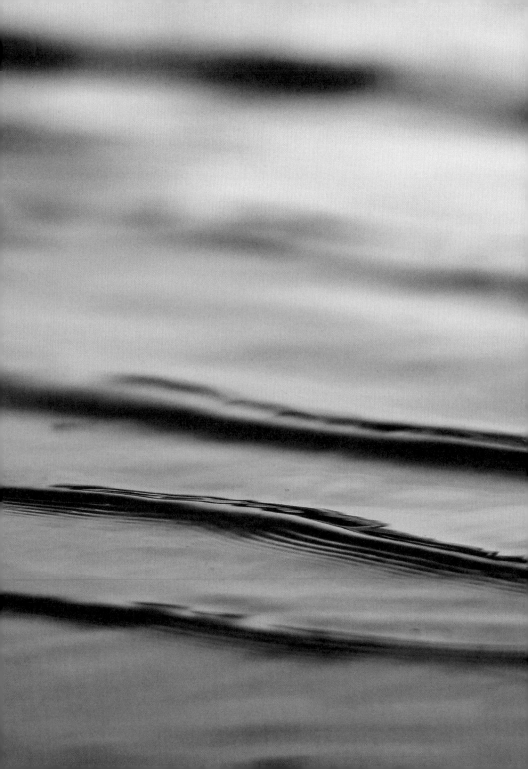

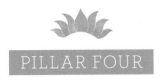

Manifestation

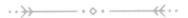

"Manifesting" is a word that's thrown around a lot in spiritual circles, but what does it really mean? Essentially, manifesting is a process of consciously creating your reality through your energy and thoughts. We're always manifesting everything that happens to us—the good things and the not so desirable things alike—which is why it's so important to be aware of how it works. There's a lot of debate and confusion around the manifestation process, however, which is why we developed our own seven-step system for manifesting. It's helped so many people create incredible things in their lives, and we're excited to share it with you before you dive into the rituals that follow!

1. *Ask with clarity.* First, it's super important to get clear on what you want and how you want to feel. You should constantly be asking yourself, "What would be my ideal outcome or situation here?" If you are ever feeling stagnant or bored or unsatisfied, start by looking at how clear you are on where you want to go from that place. Maybe you have a big-picture vision of what you want, but you haven't been specific enough about the details. It's also important to ask for what you want—starting by saying it out loud to the universe!

2. *Feel it.* Once you've gotten clarity on your desires, you must imagine how it would feel to have them and then get yourself into that energetic state as often as possible. Usually, this means raising your vibration to a frequency of happiness and joy—or, if

you can't do that right now, at least commit to feeling a little better than you are currently. Everything you want to manifest comes back to a single root cause: wanting to be happy. If you aren't feeling happy or joyful, it is just showing you that you aren't in energetic alignment with the natural state of your true self and your desires. Visualize yourself having achieved your manifestation, feel what it's like to be in that energy, and come back to this visualization as much as possible!

3. *Take action.* Start to take inspired action toward your goal that feels good. This will continue to put you into the energy of what you are manifesting and will help you elevate your vibration. We always like to ask the question, "What would my future self who has already manifested XYZ be doing right now?" What can you do *today* to move closer to your manifestation? Listen to guidance from the universe, determine what feels good from a place of empowerment, and do that.

4. *Trust.* The fourth step of our manifestation process is about cultivating the unshakable knowing that if you're in a high vibration and taking aligned action, you will always manifest what you want or something better. If you don't fully believe that you are in control of your reality, no worries; you can get there. The disbelief is just a lower state of consciousness, so as you raise your vibration and start to manifest little things, your trust and belief in the process will grow. Our rituals also help give us this trust because we have a foundation to keep our energetic vibration rising every day.

5. *Notice.* Pay attention to the signs and synchronicities from the universe that are aligned with the feeling and desires you are manifesting. Be grateful for those small wins and celebrate them! Focusing on how far you've come versus how far you still have to go will get you there even faster.

6. *Keep your vibe high.* In order to raise your vibration, you need to be clearing your subconscious mind of limiting beliefs daily and setting yourself up to feel good. For us, Kundalini yoga and meditation are the fastest, most effective ways to do this. Having a daily meditation ritual will change the game when it comes to how you feel, the quality of your thoughts, and what you are able to manifest.

7. *Release.* Finally, patience is key. Everything manifests in perfect timing. A lot of times, the universal intelligence has its own plan, and you end up manifesting things that are *way* better than what you ever could have dreamed up. If you're being patient and still not seeing any progress toward your manifestation, it comes back to energy work. How can you increase your vibration and bring in even more positive emotions? Sometimes that calls for a cleanse of sorts—letting things go that could be lowering your energy. Living your life and focusing on your happiness first will magnetize all that you ever want, even if it's taking longer than you wanted it to. Promise!

Bottom line? Manifesting really comes down to your energy, how you feel, and your mind-set. To help you on the journey, we have created rituals that you can use alongside our manifestation technique to elevate your vibration around certain kinds of manifestations: business success and opportunities, attracting and amplifying love, and becoming a magnet for miracles. If you are feeling stuck in any of these areas of your life, we want you to know that you are always just a little healing away from what you desire. You are here to learn and grow, and it's all a part of your happily ever after. Cinderella didn't find Prince Charming without a little struggle, lots of lessons, and figuring out how to stay true to herself and find happiness where she could. (Even if it was through befriending mice and singing while she mopped, there *was* a way.)

These rituals are here to guide you to where you want to be, from two Cinderellas on their way to queendom (us)—both of whom have transcended their hardships to see so many of their wildest dreams come true.

> MANIFESTING IS ONE OF MY FAVORITE TOPICS—IT WAS MY GATEWAY INTO SPIRITUALITY. IT ALL STARTED WITH READING *CHICKEN SOUP FOR THE TEENAGE SOUL* AT A YOUNG AGE AND LEARNING WHY OPTIMISM IS IMPORTANT WHEN CREATING WHAT YOU WANT. THEN, IN MY SENIOR YEAR OF COLLEGE, MY UNCLE GOT ME THE BOOK *THE SECRET,* AND I BECAME OBSESSED WITH IT. (FUN FACT: MY UNCLE'S FRIEND WAS IN THE BOOK AND THE MOVIE, WHICH MADE ME EVEN MORE OF A BELIEVER.) I WOULD WATCH THE MOVIE OVER AND OVER AGAIN WITH A BOYFRIEND AT THE TIME—WE WOULD PLAY WITH THE TECHNIQUE, AND I STARTED MANIFESTING AMAZING THINGS. OVER THE LAST FIFTEEN YEARS, I HAVE HONED MY SKILLS AND CONTINUED TO STUDY, AND HAVE BEEN BLOWN AWAY WITH WHAT I CAN CREATE. I MANIFESTED MY HUSBAND; OUR HOME; THE THREE-HOUR PAIN-FREE BIRTH OF OUR DAUGHTER; A PODCAST; A BOOK DEAL; CONNECTIONS WITH CERTAIN PEOPLE...SO MUCH! NOW, I'M FULLY CONVINCED OF THE POWER OF MANIFESTATION—AND THAT WE ALL CAN DO IT.
>
> *—Britt*

Business Success
Attract Opportunities with Ease

40–45 MINUTES

What if we told you that you are hardwired to become successful? That you get to have everything you want and become whoever you want? That the opportunities you want are already yours—they're right in front of you, just waiting for you to receive them? Would you believe us?

Well, it's true! Success is your birthright, and your thought patterns, belief systems, and habits can throw you off course and cause you to self-sabotage, especially when you're close to receiving whatever it is you've been manifesting. It's why the Elevate the Globe lifestyle is all-encompassing—it helps you develop habits and create new ways of thinking and acting that support your highest destiny.

Success can come in many shapes and forms, and we realize that everyone is starting from a different place on their journey. But no matter your current circumstances, you can begin by expanding your belief system and looking at the world through a different lens to start attracting and stepping into success with confidence and ease. Successful people understand they have to change their thoughts and habits to receive the things they don't already have. It will look different for everyone, but the commonality is that it's possible for everyone to attain their version of success—and they can have fun doing it.

We're so excited to share this ritual with you because you're going to forge a connection with the planet of luck, knowledge, and expansion: Jupiter. You'll strengthen your nervous system to handle whatever success is coming your way and remove obstacles like anger and frustration that keep you from receiving all that you want.

Are you ready to expand into that new you and open the floodgates to all the manifestations that have been waiting for you? Let's get started!

Gather

- Yoga mat, meditation cushion, or chair.

- Journal and pen.

- Ingredients for the Raw Cacao Latte.

Tune In

Come down onto your mat, sitting in a cross-legged position. Alternatively, you can sit in a chair with shoes off and both feet flat on the ground. Rub your palms together and bring them into your heart center in a prayer position. Begin your ritual by tuning in with the "Adi Mantra"—"Ong Namo Guroo Dayv Namo"—three times.

Play the mantra "Gobinday Mukunday" as much as you can—at the office, in your car, while you're at the gym. This mantra powerfully clears your subconscious mind of all the unhelpful patterns and beliefs that are creating your current reality. It's said to help you bust through blocks—some of which you probably didn't even know you had. We love the version by Snatam Kaur on the album Prem. *(Check it out on the Spotify playlist that accompanies this book!)*

Warm-Up

We're going to start with Life-Nerve Stretch. This exercise will help keep your spine long and healthy, plus it will release muscle tension and resistance in the body and the mind. It will help you remain calm. The most successful business people make decisions from a calm and collected place—this way you're able to clearly and confidently connect to your intuition.

Still sitting down, bring your legs straight out in front of you. Start by taking a deep breath in and stretching your arms over your head. As you exhale, bring your arms forward to grab your toes. If you can, wrap your index and middle fingers behind your big toes and press your thumbs into the toenails. You can also hold your ankles or shins instead.

Stay in this position and breathe deeply through the nose.

Close the eyes and continue for two minutes.

To end, inhale with a flat back and exhale, bringing your nose to your knees. Slowly come back up to Easy Pose (a cross-legged position).

Meditation

This meditation is called Hast Kriya, and it will connect you with the planet Jupiter.[26] It's said that if you practice this meditation for twenty-two minutes a day, you can totally remove anger and obnoxious behaviors from your personality—things that can keep you from manifesting success. You can completely change how you respond to the world and how it responds back to you.

Posture + Mudra + Mantra. Extend your Jupiter (index) fingers of both hands. Lock the other fingers down with your thumbs. Time the following movements with the chant "Sat Naam Whaa-hay Guroo," which is the mantra that connects you to Jupiter. We recommend listening to the version by Jagjit Singh called "Sat Nam Wahe Guru #2," found on YouTube, but you can also just chant the mantra silently in your mind.

Movement. Touch your Jupiter fingers to the floor on either side of you on "*Sat.*"

Touch your Jupiter fingers together over the top of your head on "*Naam.*"

Touch your Jupiter fingers to the floor on either side of you on "*Sat.*"

Touch your Jupiter fingers together over the top of your head on "*Naam.*"

Touch your Jupiter fingers to the floor on either side of you on "*Whaa-hay.*"

Touch your Jupiter fingers together over the top of your head on "*Guroo.*"

Touch your Jupiter fingers to the floor on either side of you on "*Whaa-hay.*"

Touch your Jupiter fingers together over the top of your head on "*Guroo.*"

Time. Continue for twenty-two minutes.

Okay, we know what you're thinking—twenty-two minutes is a really *long time to meditate each day. But it's a small (and exciting!) investment in your future to adjust your energy, remove obstacles, and manifest your desires. The twenty-two minutes will fly by, and we guarantee you'll have fun with this meditation. It's kind of like dancing with Jupiter, the planet of expansion and luck!*

Seal your practice with Sat Naam. Bring your hands together in Prayer Pose in front of your heart. Inhale deeply and either chant or say out loud "Sat Naam," which means "truth is my essence."

Visualization + Affirmation

Sitting in silence after your mediation, allow yourself to relax and surrender into the moment. Breathe long and deep and visualize yourself receiving opportunities you've been manifesting, no matter how small or big they are. What does it feel like to have this type of success? Study the version of you that's receiving it with open arms. Repeat this affirmation to end:

> *I step out of the way and allow myself to receive all the opportunities that are meant for me.*

Journal

Write down what you need to do today to become the future version of yourself that has next-level success. Who are you? How do you spend your day? What kinds of changes do you need to focus on and begin making?

Nourishment

Swap your daily, heavy dose of caffeine with a cup of raw cacao. Cacao is one of the most high-vibrational foods on the planet and will help give you that extra energy boost without leading to a caffeine crash at 3:00 p.m. Just one small serving of cacao strengthens the neural pathways and triggers the brain to release endorphins that make you feel oh so good.

RAW CACAO LATTE

Prep time: 10 minutes
Makes 1 serving

1 cup water or plant-based milk

2–3 tablespoons of raw cacao powder (Raw, organic, unsweetened, and fair-trade preferred so you don't get all the sugars and fillers and you know it's ethically sourced.)

>> Warm up your water or plant-based milk in a pan until you hear the first pop, then remove from the heat. Using a whisk, beat half of the cacao into the water until it's completely dissolved. Heat up once more until the cacao reaches your desired temperature. Remove from the heat and fill your cup halfway. Whisk the remaining cacao powder into the remaining water in the pan so it becomes frothy. Once dissolved, add your frothed cacao mixture into your cup.

You can spice up your cacao using a dash of vanilla extract or nutmeg during the heating stage and sweeten with maple syrup.

> ❝❞
>
> NOTHING LEFT TO DO BUT ENJOY YOURSELF AND ALL THE SUCCESS ON ITS WAY TO YOU! OPPORTUNITIES OF YOUR WILDEST DREAMS FALL AT YOUR DOORSTEP TODAY. WHAT AN EXCITING LIFE YOU'RE LIVING, AND IT'S EXPANDING EVERY DAY!
>
> *—XO, B+T*

Attract and Amplify Love

*Magnetize Your Soul Mate, Find a Twin
Flame, or Spice Up Existing Love*

35–40 MINUTES

If you are fed up with finding love—or you're in a relationship that's less than satisfying—you might be skeptical about this ritual. Maybe you're ready to give up now and hand this stupid book back to whoever gave it to you (a pushy mother who says you must be married by thirty-five, perhaps, or the annoying coworker who tries to get you to go on double dates all the time). Or maybe you bought it after yoga in a fleeting moment of hope, but you've since come back to the cruel reality of swipe-lefts and apps made for cheating on your spouse. Believe us, we get it. But before you close the book, hear us out.

Despite what you may believe, love is not about finding the perfect partner or being in the picture-perfect relationship. It's about healing insecurities and amplifying your divine essence. Most people unhappy in love are looking for security in someone else, and we can tell you now, no one can guarantee that. The good thing is that there's another way, and it starts with doing some inner dirty work (yes, *more*) and really looking at your relationship with your own security. You must be whole within yourself to attract what you want in a partnership because our lovers are our mirrors, reflecting where we can love ourselves more to then increase intimacy, partnership, and deep love for another. When you're in love with being alive in your own skin, an authentic relationship is just the cherry on top of your already very delicious, ice-cream-sundae existence.

It's time to go deeper, clarify your true worth, and learn what it means to purify yourself with love. This ritual will help you let go of the fear, insecurity, pain, and judgment overpowering your love muscle, allowing you to fall in love with yourself and become a magnet for the relationship you desire. Because the truth is, love is worth it. It can take everything—including possibilities for you and your manifestations in this incarnation—to a whole new level.

Gather

- Yoga mat, meditation cushion, or chair.
- Emerald or jade crystal if you are in a relationship or rose quartz if you are manifesting love.
- Rose oil, with almond or coconut oil to act as a carrier oil.
- Rose water spray.
- Journal and pen.
- A green apple.

Journal

Upon waking, write down the first thing you think about so you can become more conscious of the thoughts that are running through your mind. If it's negative, write a truer, kinder, or better thought next to it. This will help your unconscious mind shift these ideas about yourself, your partner, or others to a more loving place. Lastly, write a little love letter to yourself—anything that will make you smile.

Tune In

Come down onto your mat, sitting in a cross-legged position. Alternatively, you can sit in a chair with shoes off and both feet flat on the ground. Rub your palms together and bring them into your heart center in a prayer position. Begin your ritual by tuning in with the "Adi Mantra"—"Ong Namo Guroo Dayv Namo"—three times.

Mantra

Play the "So Purkh" mantra and really listen to it as you are doing the following warm-up and meditation. This mantra was given to women by Guru Ram Das, the fourth guru of the Sikhs, to help them raise the vibration of the men in their lives—but it can be used to help *any* partner live up to their full potential. You can also use it to attract an aligned partner if you haven't met them yet. We love the version called "So Purkh (Gurmukhi Recitation)" by Nirinjan Kaur Khalsa, found on the Spotify playlist that accompanies this book.

If you want to take this part of the ritual to another level, sit and chant "So Purkh" eleven times a day for forty days straight. This is said to manifest God in physical male form before the eyes of a woman, but in our mind, it applies to everyone who's trying to manifest a partnership, regardless of gender. You can even listen to the mantra while you sleep to help align you with this energy. We've heard some crazy stories about people calling in partners using this mantra!

Warm-Up

We'll start by coming into Ustrasana, or Camel Pose, to direct the energy we are cultivating toward the heart center. This will allow expansion and brightness to activate physically and emotionally.

Come up so you are standing on your knees and shins, torso upright. Place your hands on your hips and draw your abdomen in to support your lower back. Relax your shoulder blades down and press them gently into your back. Inhale and lift your chest. You can keep your hands on your hips and lean back a little bit or release your hands down to hold on to your heels. If it's comfortable for your neck, drop your head back. For both options, practice long, deep breathing, expanding the stomach and heart center as you inhale and contracting the abdomen in toward the spine on the exhale.

Continue breathing in this position for one to two minutes—you can spend more time in the pose as you develop your practice. After you are done, take a big inhale and hold it for a couple of seconds. Then exhale and very slowly bring yourself back to a neutral spine. Shake out your hands and legs and grab a sip of water.

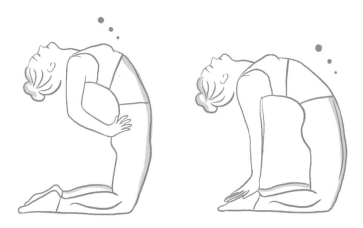

Movement + Meditation

Next, we will go into a powerful three-part meditation to open the heart, create a positive relationship with yourself, release fear, and purify you with love.[27]

PART 1

This exercise is called Reverse Adi Shakti Kriya. You are mentally and hypnotically blessing yourself to affect and correct the magnetic field. It is said that doing this exercise will hurt if you have a lot of anger. Self-help is very difficult for those who are angry. After doing this exercise for five minutes, your muscles may start hurting if your diet needs cleaning up. The taste in your mouth will change if you are breathing correctly.

Posture. Sit in Easy Pose with a straight spine and hold your right palm six to nine inches above the top center of your head. The right palm faces down, blessing you. This self-blessing corrects the aura. The left elbow is bent with the upper arm near the rib cage. The forearm and hand point upward. The left palm faces forward and blesses the world.

Eyes. The eyes are closed, turned down, and focused at the lunar center—in the middle of the chin.

Breath. Breathe long, slow, and deep with a feeling of self-affection. Try to bring the breath to one breath per minute: inhale for twenty seconds, hold for twenty seconds, exhale for twenty seconds. If your current lung capacity doesn't allow this timing, reduce each part to ten, ten, ten or five, five, five.

Time. Continue for eleven minutes. Then inhale deeply and move slowly and directly into position for part 2.

PART 2

This exercise will benefit everything between the neck and navel. It will give strength to the heart and will open up the heart center.

Posture. Extend your arms straight out in front, parallel to the ground, palms facing down. Stretch out to your maximum.

Eyes. The eyes are closed and focused at the lunar center in the middle of the chin.

Breath. The breath is long, slow, and deep.

Time. Continue for three minutes. Then inhale deeply and move slowly and directly into position for part 3.

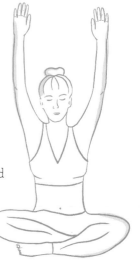

PART 3

Posture. Stretch your arms straight up with the palms facing forward. There is no bend in the elbows.

Eyes. The eyes are closed and focused at the lunar center in the middle of the chin.

Breath. The breath continues to be long, slow, and deep.

Time. Continue for three minutes.

To end. Inhale and hold your breath for ten seconds while you stretch your arms upward (try to stretch so much that your buttocks are lifted) and tighten all the muscles of your body. Exhale. Repeat this sequence two more times.

Come on to your back for a minute to rest and normalize your breath. Hold whatever crystal you are working with or place it on your heart center to align yourself with the vibration of love.

Seal your practice with Sat Naam. Bring your hands together in Prayer Pose in front of your heart. Inhale deeply and either chant or say out loud "Sat Naam," which means "truth is my essence."

If you're short on time, you can cut the duration of each posture in half. But we highly recommend doing it for the full seventeen minutes whenever possible!

Visualization + Affirmation

After the meditation, sit and visualize either the most amazing things about your current partner or the things that are important to you in a future partner. It can be anything positive you can think of—why you fell in love, their strengths, how they make you feel good—and doesn't have to be something you're experiencing yet. It can be how you *want* to feel.

Next, visualize what your partner (or future partner) loves about you. Get clear on how they are getting what they need from the relationship and how you make them feel good.

Now say, "Universe, amplify that by a hundred times," and feel the energy amplifying.

Repeat this affirmation either mentally or out loud:

> *I am becoming more secure with who I am every day, and I am finding more love and acceptance with myself and my life. I am amplifying the love in my life to unimaginable levels, and I'm doing it for me.*

Self-Care

Mist your face with some rose water spray. Then, put two or three drops of rose oil into a carrier oil (we recommend coconut or almond oil) and give yourself a quick back and neck massage while sending yourself tons of love.

Nourishment

Forget keeping the doctor away—we believe a green apple a day brings all the love to the yard...ha! But seriously, we want you to dance your way into the kitchen and eat a green apple on an empty stomach. Why? Any whole, green foods are going to help balance and open the heart chakra. Plus, green apples have tons of benefits—they are a rich source of metabolism-boosting fiber and antioxidants. Since we learned this, we eat one almost every day, and we are excited for you to try it for forty days for this ritual!

> ❝❞
>
> YOU ARE INCREDIBLY SPECIAL, THERE IS TRULY NO ONE ELSE LIKE YOU IN THE WORLD, AND HELLO, THAT IS WHY YOU ARE HERE! **YOU DESERVE TO LOVE YOURSELF LIKE CRAZY AND GIVE AND RECEIVE LOVE,** AND WE ARE ROOTING YOU ON AND SENDING TONS OF LOVE YOUR WAY TODAY AND ALWAYS, BABE.
>
> *—XO, B+T*

Magnet for Miracles
Manifest Specific Desires

25-35 MINUTES

When you aren't clear on what you want—step 1 of our manifesting process!—it's often because your subconscious mind is filled with past memories, traumas, untrue stories, and old experiences. This is especially true in the Aquarian Age of information, a time when we have so much going into these noggins of ours day in and day out. If we don't make an effort to clean out our subconscious minds, life can become a hot mess *fast*.

If you are new to the subconscious mind, it is simply the place where the things we are not conscious of get stored away, but those things are still present and drive our actions. It is basically made up of what spills over from the conscious mind and is filed away so you are no longer conscious of it, but it is hanging out, still there. That is why it is so important to clear it out—because all that past junk affects our energy, and our energy is what drives our manifestations! Make sense?

No matter what your past has been or where you are at now, you can absolutely become a magnet for miracles and manifest specific desires and get really good at it. It starts with clarity and comes down to elevating your energy and cultivating the feeling of what it is that you want so it can be delivered to you on a silver (or gold—be clear!) platter by a butler if you so choose!

This morning ritual is a way to clear out the garbage in your head and create space to magnetize your desires to you—rather than chasing after them at the expense of your health and happiness, as is the norm in many cultures. We aren't willing to suffer from burnout and stress-related health issues in pursuit of our dreams, and you don't have to either!

Gather

- Yoga mat, meditation cushion, or chair.

- Clear quartz crystal. This stone is great for manifesting, as it amplifies your energetic vibration. Keep it in your lap during meditation, near your bed while you're sleeping, or even put it under your pillow to amplify your aura all night long.

- Litsea oil. Before you tune in, put a few drops of litsea oil—aka "the oil for manifesting"—into some almond oil and apply it to your wrists and palms. Rub your palms together, hold them up to your nose, and take a few deep breaths in, smelling the uplifting citrus scent. The vibration of litsea grounds your manifestations to bring them into reality.

- Journal and pen.

- Rainbow Chia Seed Pudding. We recommend prepping this recipe in advance.

Affirmation

As soon as you wake up, think or say out loud:

I am a ridiculously powerful manifestor making the world a better place just by being here! Today I am focused on feeling great. I am so excited to manifest incredible things today because today is a gift that is only here once.

You can even set this as the message that pops up when your phone alarm goes off. Get all Jerry Maguire on yourself and feel that energy amping up.

66 99

I HAVE BEEN WORKING WITH THE LAW OF ATTRACTION FOR A WHILE NOW AND LOVE TO PLAY WITH IT AND TEST THINGS OUT AND HAVE FUN WITH ATTRACTING THINGS. I DID IT FOR OUR HOUSE. I HAD A PICTURE OF IT ON A PINTEREST VISION BOARD AND DID ALL THE STEPS TO MANIFEST IT. WHEN ALMOST FIFTY PEOPLE PUT OFFERS DOWN AND A PAY-IN-CASH OFFER WAS ACCEPTED BY THE OWNER, I STILL TRUSTED IT WAS OURS. I USED THE LAW OF ACTION AND WAS INSPIRED TO WRITE A LETTER AND HAVE OUR REALTOR CALL THE SELLERS. THEY GAVE US THE BACK-UP OFFER POSITION. THEN, THE FIRST CASH OFFER FELL THROUGH, AND WE GOT IT!

SAME THING WITH HAVING FAST LABORS AND BIRTHS FOR BOTH OF MY DAUGHTERS. FOR MY FIRST DAUGHTER, EVEREST, I HEARD ABOUT A WOMAN WHO GAVE BIRTH IN THREE HOURS, AND I TOLD MY MIDWIVES THAT'S WHAT I WANTED—EVEN THOUGH THEY LOVINGLY LAUGHED AT ME AND SAID IT WAS VERY UNLIKELY. I BEGAN MANIFESTING A BEAUTIFUL, NATURAL, FAST, PAIN-FREE, OUT-OF-HOSPITAL BIRTH, AND THAT'S EXACTLY WHAT HAPPENED. I HAD EVEREST IN JUST AROUND THREE HOURS, AND I WANTED TO BEAT THAT FOR MY SECOND DAUGHTER, FINNLYN. I DELIVERED HER IN ONE HOUR AND FIFTEEN MINUTES! BOTH WERE BEAUTIFUL, NATURAL, AND SPIRITUAL EXPERIENCES! **YOU CAN MANIFEST ANYTHING YOU WANT, AND IT BECOMES A FUN GAME TO PLAY WITH WHEN YOU GET IN THE ENERGY OF IT AND TRUST IT WILL ALWAYS BE WHAT YOU WANT OR SOMETHING BETTER!**

—Britt

Tune In

Come down onto your mat, sitting in a cross-legged position. Alternatively, you can sit in a chair with shoes off and both feet flat on the ground. Rub your palms together and bring them into your heart center in a prayer position. Begin your ritual by tuning in with the "Adi Mantra"—"Ong Namo Guroo Dayv Namo"—three times.

Warm-Up

We'll start by clearing the subconscious with Ego Eradicator: a posture and breathwork that balances the ego, which is the driver of a lot of defensive action from the subconscious mind.[28] This warm-up is also going to bring the hemispheres of the brain to alertness and consolidate the magnetic field, which will bring you clarity and amp up your magnetism.

Posture. This exercise can be done in Easy Pose (cross-legged position) or with knees bent and your feet under your bum in Rock Pose. Raise the arms up to a sixty-degree angle. Keep the elbows straight and the shoulders down. Pull your chin in and down so your spine is straight and aligned, in what we call Neck Lock. Curl the fingertips onto the pads of the palms at the base of the fingers. Thumbs are stretched back, pointing toward each other.

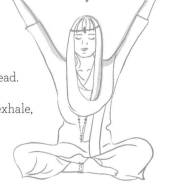

Eyes. Eyes are closed.

Mental focus. Turn your attention above the head.

Breath. Do the Breath of Fire (inhale and exhale, equal in strength and length, through the nose; allow the navel point (the energy center located two to three inches below the belly button) to move with the breath, expanding on the inhale, contracting on the exhale) or long, deep breathing (slowly inhaling through the nose, expanding your belly out, and exhaling slowly and completely out the nose while contracting the stomach in) if you are on the first three days of your moon cycle or pregnant.

Time. Continue for one to three minutes.

To end. Inhale deeply and bring the arms overhead with the thumb tips touching. Open the fingers, exhale, and relax the arms down.

Mantra

Now think about the feeling you cultivated in the previous step of the ritual and listen to "Ek Ong Kaar Satgur Parsaad." You can find it on the Spotify playlist that accompanies this book. It's called "Expand into Intuitive Knowing (Ek Ong Kar Sat Gur Prasad)" by Jai-Jagdeesh. This is the only Kundalini mantra that comes with a warning!

> This is such a powerful and creative mantra that you must watch your thoughts and actions after you chant it. You will be in such a state of manifestation that your thoughts will accelerate into being. Luckily, the energy within the mantra itself will help you switch your thoughts to the positive. It takes your own negative thought, stops it in its tracks, and reverses it into positivity. A thought rides into your consciousness to be processed with "Ek Ong Kaar Satgur Parsaad" and comes out pure with "Satgur Parsaad Ek Ong Kaar."[29]

Sing along with it for one to three minutes!

Movement + Meditation

Shake out your hands and legs and grab a sip of water—we're about to go into a powerful, three-part meditation to clear the mind of distracting thoughts and

attachments with the Beam and Create Your Future Meditation.[30] It will cultivate tremendous capacity and creativity that is focused and beaming. The best
way to practice this is on an empty stomach; also, be sure to drink a lot of
liquids throughout the day afterward.

Posture. Sit in a cross-legged position. Stretch the
spine up and become very still.

Eye focus. Eyes are closed.

Mudra. Rest the hands on the knees in Gyan
Mudra, with the tips of the thumbs and index
fingers touching and the rest of the fingers
out straight.

PART 1

Take a single, deep, long inhale through a rounded mouth, as if you're sipping
through a straw. Close the mouth and exhale through the nose, slowly and
completely. Continue for seven minutes.

PART 2

Inhale and hold the breath comfortably. As you suspend the breath in, meditate on zero. Think in this way: *All is zero; I am zero; each thought is zero; my
pain is zero; that problem is zero; that illness is zero.*

Meditate on all negative, emotional, mental, and physical conditions and situations. As each thing crosses the mind, bring it to zero—a single point of light,
a small, insignificant nonexistence.

Exhale and repeat. Breathe in a comfortable rhythm. Continue for seven
minutes.

PART 3

Think of the quality or condition you most desire for your complete happiness and growth. Summarize it in a single word like "wealth," "health," "relationship," "guidance," "knowledge," "luck." It has to be one word. Lock on that word and thought. Visualize facets of it. Inhale and suspend the breath as you beam the thought in a continuous stream. Lock onto it. Relax the breath as needed. Continue for five minutes.

To end. Inhale and move the shoulders, arms, and spine any way you feel called to. Then stretch the arms up, spread the fingers wide, and breathe deeply a few times.

Seal your practice with Sat Naam. Bring your hands together in Prayer Pose in front of your heart. Inhale deeply and either chant or say out loud "Sat Naam," which means "truth is my essence."

Write the word you came up with in your journal to really ground it in the physical.

Journal + Visualization

Get clear on how you want to feel today and what you want to manifest as a result of that feeling. Then, write those future manifestations in the past tense, as if they already happened. Example: "It was so amazing to travel to Positano, Italy, and be pampered with my love. The food was incredible, the water was so clear, and it was the most invigorating and rejuvenating trip. I can't wait to go back!"

Finish by writing "And so it is," and take a moment to visualize how it looked for you.

Write down different things for each of the forty days you perform this ritual. They can be small or big, but after you write down a desire, don't ask for it again. Release it and trust it is coming in perfect timing.

Nourishment

Head to the kitchen (while you picture yourself walking toward the manifested kitchen of your dreams) to eat your Rainbow Chia Seed Pudding. This recipe is filled with omega-3 fatty acids that help decrease inflammation and improve brain function and clarity.[31] Its rainbow toppings help balance the chakras to amplify the amazing energy you just created! We recommend batch-prepping this recipe in advance to save time, as it needs to sit for a while before you eat it.

RAINBOW CHIA SEED PUDDING

Prep time: 5 minutes (plus at least 2 hours in the fridge to get firm)
Makes 1 serving

 2 tablespoons chia seeds

 ½ cup almond or coconut milk

 Toppings:

 Walnuts

 1 tablespoon almond butter

 Rainbow-colored fruits: strawberries, oranges, pineapple, kiwi, blueberries, blackberries (We recommend choosing organic, local, and in-season fruits. You can switch out these options with different fruits of the same color if needed.)

>> Put the chia seeds and milk in a mason jar and mix until the chia seeds are well incorporated. Let the mixture settle and mix it well again. Then, close the mason jar and put it in the fridge for two hours to seven days. Add toppings and enjoy!

If you need some extra grounding, take your shoes off and walk in the grass, dirt, or sand or on concrete today. You have cleared and created a lot of energy for your manifestations, and we want to make sure you are present and grounded, which is key to experiencing them physically.

> 66 99
>
> YOU HAVE TASTED THE RAINBOW AND ARE SO CLEAR THAT PEOPLE MIGHT BE ABLE TO SEE RIGHT THROUGH YOU. YOU MIGHT FLY TO WORK TODAY...OR TO THE BEACH OR ITALY OR ANYWHERE ELSE YOU WANT TO MANIFEST. WE ARE SO EXCITED FOR YOU AS YOU COCREATE YOUR LIFE WITH THE UNIVERSE AND BRING MASSIVE LOVE TO THE PLANET.
>
> *—XO, B+T*

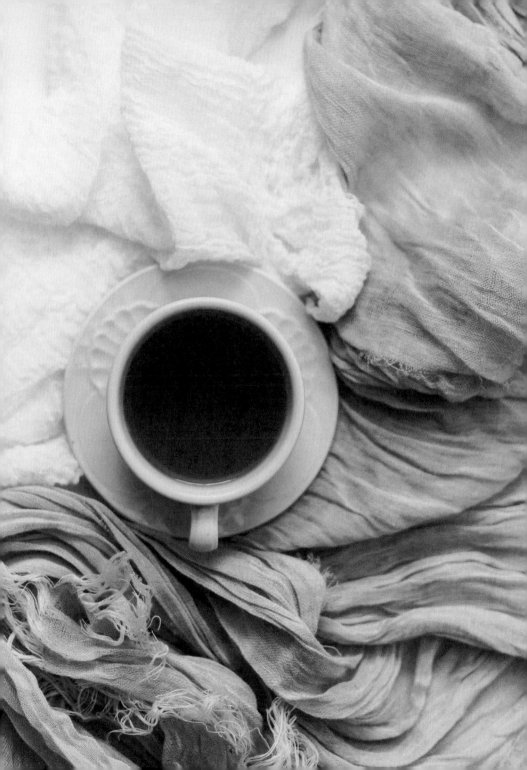

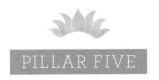

Self-Love and Self-Care

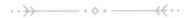

We believe in celebrating self-love every single day by taking time to connect with the truth of who we really are—not who social media tells us we should be. Loving and caring for the self is an inside *and* an outside job. It's just as much about being deeply committed to nurturing your inner world as it is about your Sunday night face masks, ritual baths, and monthly massages. A focus on both will leave you feeling like you're emanating radiance and beauty from the inside out.

Oftentimes our inner world gets overlooked because it can be confronting to look at what's going on inside our minds, bodies, and souls. It takes courage, strength, and discipline to develop this inner relationship with the self, especially if we don't like what we see at first. But without this deep connection to our inner worlds, we can become disconnected from the source of love, joy, and happiness that is within us and always available to us.

Self-love is especially crucial in this Aquarian Age, when we're becoming more and more disconnected from ourselves and each other. Loneliness is an epidemic that's influenced by the very same technology that allows us to connect instantly to someone across the globe, although it's not the defining factor. A study in 2018 surveyed twenty thousand US adults, and around 46 percent of people said they always feel alone or left out, with Gen Z reportedly the loneliest of all the generations.[32] Never before has it been more important, if not mandatory, to have a deep and vibrant relationship with yourself.

When you feel disconnected in any way, in any area of your life—your career, relationship, or health—you are not connected to yourself and the energy of love that resides within you. Feeling separate, lonely, or misunderstood is a sign that you are more tuned in to fear than to love. The disconnect can happen from past parental or societal programming, unprocessed grief or trauma, or different ideas you've picked up along the way. If you ever feel lost or off-track, start by returning to the relationship you have with yourself. This approach never fails because our outer reality is a reflection of our inner vibration. It takes a lot of unlearning to get back to a love vibration, but you can do it—and it can be fun!

Healing the energy that has been keeping you disconnected, developing a strong self-concept, and understanding who you are at a soul level is what helps you care for and fall in love with yourself. When you know yourself and understand how to take care of your inner needs, your self-confidence and self-esteem skyrocket. This type of lovefest with your true self gives you power.

We created the rituals in this section to help you develop a strong and deep relationship with yourself during challenging times. From transforming addictions and healing from heartbreak to looking and feeling youthful at any age, these practices can help you connect to that inner love that is always there like a lighthouse, guiding you back into your own safe harbor. You'll be shining brighter as you amp up your radiance from the inside out.

Addiction Rehab
Heal the Addiction Urge

18-22 MINUTES

There are many different addictions we can pick up as coping mechanisms, all of which are essentially ways to disconnect from reality and keep from feeling much at all. You may just want to numb out, which might look like checking your phone a hundred times a day, getting sucked into that low-vibe reality show yet again, or something a lot more serious. Recent studies show the most common substance addictions are cigarettes, alcohol, marijuana, and painkillers or prescription drugs.[33] Then, there are behavioral addictions to things like food—about 20 percent of people have a food addiction, and the most habit-forming foods are pizza and chocolate—gambling, pornography, sex, codependent relationships, overworking, shopping, the internet, or plastic surgery.[34] There are also much more subtle addictions, such as clinging to ideas or certain thoughts, looking for belonging outside of yourself, hanging out with people who don't make you feel good, procrastinating, getting approval, controlling how others view you, blaming others for your misery, obsessive thinking, defending, explaining, resisting, withdrawing...the list goes on. If you are addicted to something outside yourself, you aren't connected to the truth and magic that everything you need is inside of you.

If you aren't sure whether you are addicted to something, ask yourself if you want to stop but feel like you can't. Before you can heal an addiction, you have to be aware of it.

In terms of the energetics of addiction, which is what we always examine to get to the root of the issue, we have to look at the chakras, the main energy centers in our bodies. According to Tibetan master Djwhal Khul, addictions are an indication of a blocked heart chakra. When we manifest anything on this physical plane, it originates as information coming in through the crown and third-eye chakras. Then, that information moves down the energy centers and is birthed as an action through the sacral chakra. But when the heart chakra is blocked—the one that acts as a bridge between the physical and spiritual worlds—we can't receive the spiritual energy that's trying to come in and guide us.

We create addictions to try to deal with the pain that caused the blocked heart chakra in the first place. This pain is usually connected to an imbalanced root chakra—caused by a real or perceived life-threatening trauma or a lack of security and safety—or an imbalanced solar plexus, which stems from traumatic events that lower self-esteem and feelings of empowerment. If this trauma is not dealt with when it occurs, it can move into grief and turn into addiction as a coping mechanism.

If you are new to chakras or find this confusing, don't worry! The main thing to realize is if you are addicted to something, you can heal and release it using energy work. (You should also seek help from a professional, especially if you're dealing with substance abuse or a serious behavioral addiction.) This ritual won't just help you let go of existing addictions—it'll also help you heal challenging events as they come so they don't impact your energetic flow. You will be able to handle the ups and downs of life much more gracefully and prevent the inherited cycle of addiction that might be in your family from passing to future generations.

The silver lining is addictions can be some of our greatest paths for empowerment and can allow us to find massive "gifts from the garbage"! So let's start to get a little dirty, uncovering and rediscovering the badass, unlimited potential that is waiting for you on the other side! Are you in?

> **66 99**
>
> I WAS ADDICTED TO SO MUCH: ALCOHOL, CIGARETTES, CODEPENDENT RELATIONSHIPS, AND EVEN DRUGS FOR A PERIOD OF TIME. I MOSTLY USED THESE THINGS SOCIALLY, AND I WAS STILL ABLE TO DO VERY WELL IN MY CORPORATE CAREER AND HIDE MY HABITS FROM A LOT OF FAMILY AND FRIENDS, SO I DIDN'T REALLY THINK OF THEM AS ADDICTIONS. BUT THEY REALLY STARTED TO AFFECT MY MENTAL WELL-BEING. I WAS NOT HAPPY, AND I WAS NUMBING EVERYTHING. AFTER A BREAKUP, I HIT ROCK BOTTOM WITH IT ALL. EVEN THE ADDICTIONS WEREN'T ENOUGH TO COVER UP THE PAIN I WAS FEELING. I THANKFULLY FELL INTO A KUNDALINI YOGA CLASS AND STARTED PRACTICING EVERY WEEK. THE MEDITATION IN THIS RITUAL WAS THE FIRST THIRTY-DAY MEDITATION I DID, THANKS TO MY TEACHER COLIN KIM. WITHOUT HAVING TO FORCE ANYTHING, I NATURALLY STARTED TO BE LESS ATTRACTED TO CIGARETTES, DRUGS, AND DRINKING. SOON, I DIDN'T EVEN WANT THEM ANYMORE. SO MUCH OF THE ENERGY OF ADDICTION WAS RELEASED, AND I OWE IT TO THE PRACTICES IN THIS RITUAL!
>
> *—Britt*

Gather

- Yoga mat, meditation cushion, or chair.

- Staurolite or clear quartz crystals. Staurolite is a mineral that resembles a cross and helps you let go of habits, relationships, and situations that do not serve you. Use clear quartz in tandem to amplify the staurolite's power and to help you renew yourself. We'd suggest wearing either of these stones or keeping them with you throughout your day. You can also just use one or the other—it's not necessary to have both, but the combination is very powerful!

- Eucalyptus oil. Before you begin, rub a drop of eucalyptus oil into your palms. Place your hands over your face and deeply inhale. This will help your nervous system relax.

- Ingredients for No-More-Cravings Millet Porridge.

Tune In

Come down onto your mat, sitting in a cross-legged position. Alternatively, you can sit in a chair with shoes off and both feet flat on the ground. Rub your palms together and bring them into your heart center in a prayer position. Begin your ritual by tuning in with the "Adi Mantra"—"Ong Namo Guroo Dayv Namo"—three times.

Mantra

During the breathwork portion of this ritual, play the "Saa Taa Naa Maa" mantra—the Kundalini yoga mantra to break habits and addictions. We love the version by Mirabai Ceiba, which you can find on the Spotify playlist we made to accompany this book!

Saa = Infinity, Taa = Life, Naa = Death, Maa = Rebirth

4-Part Energizing Breath Meditation

Next, we'll do a powerful breathwork practice to strengthen the navel point. This powerful energy center is located two to three inches below the belly button, and it's where thousands of nerve endings come together in the body. Kundalini yoga considers this the balance point in the body, and you want to stimulate and align this center of gravity to give you strength, energy, and willpower.

According to yogic science, many common addictions—especially smoking, drugs, and alcohol—are related to a lack of the fire element within. Navel breathing, especially the 4-Part Breath, explained below, gives you the fire energy you need. As you create that fire energy inside of you, you become less reliant on the addiction to create it for you.[35]

Commitment is key to releasing any addiction, and a strong navel center is necessary when it comes to keeping your commitments to yourself. So let's get into it!

Posture. Sit up straight. Place the palms together at the heart center with fingers pointing up. If you press the hands very hard and do it vigorously, one minute will recharge you, and you will get so much more out of this portion of the ritual.

Eyes. Focus at the brow point with eyelids lightly closed.

Breath. Inhale, breaking the breath into four equal sniffs, filling the lungs completely on the fourth. As you exhale, release the breath equally in that same four-part equal breathing pattern, emptying the lungs on the fourth breath. On each part of both the inhale and the exhale, pull the navel point toward the spine. (The stronger you pump the navel, the more energy you will generate.) One full breath cycle (in and out) takes about seven to eight seconds.

If your mind has a lot of anxiety or confusion, mentally chant the mantra "Saa Taa Naa Maa" on the inhale and the exhale—one syllable of the mantra for each of the four parts of the breath.

Time. Continue for two to three minutes.

To end. Inhale deeply and press the palms together with force for ten to fifteen seconds. Create tension in the whole body by pressing as hard as you can. Hold the breath as long as possible. Exhale powerfully and repeat the inhale. Hold the breath and press the hands together. Exhale, relax, and allow the tension in the body to vanish.

If you need to rest, immediately lie on your back with eyes closed and relax for two to five minutes. Take a few deep breaths, stretch, and you will be ready for action.

This breathwork will relax you and release fatigue at the same time. It can be used whenever you are craving the object of your addiction and is also great to do between 3:00 and 4:00 p.m. to prevent the post-lunch dippidy-dip in energy!

Movement

To continue activating the energy at the navel point, come on to your back for the amazingly powerful Alternate Leg Lifts. (An added benefit is some serious ab toning!)

Place your hands on the floor, palms facing down, or under your hips if you need extra support for your lower back. Inhale slowly as you pull the low belly in and lift your left leg to ninety degrees, toes pointed toward the ceiling. Exhale slowly as you lower the leg down.

Alternate left and right legs, and continue for three minutes.

To end, pull both legs up to ninety degrees and take a deep, powerful inhale. Hold the breath for five to ten seconds, then slowly release your legs down to

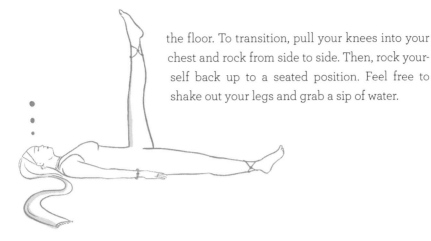

the floor. To transition, pull your knees into your chest and rock from side to side. Then, rock yourself back up to a seated position. Feel free to shake out your legs and grab a sip of water.

Meditation

The Meditation for Healing Addictions triggers certain points in the brain that are said to free you from the addiction pattern.

Posture. Sit in a cross-legged position and create a Neck Lock (called *Jalandhar Bandh*) by sitting tall, straightening the spine, and tucking your chin slightly down and back so your neck is totally straight.

Mudra. Make fists with both hands, keeping the thumbs free, and extend the thumbs straight. Place the thumbs on the temples, finding the niche where the thumbs just fit.

Lock the back molars together and keep the lips closed. Keeping the teeth pressed together throughout, alternately squeeze the molars tightly and then release the pressure. A muscle will move in rhythm under the thumbs. Feel it massage the thumbs and apply a firm pressure with the hands.

Eyes. Keep the eyes closed and focus on the point in between the eyebrows.

Mantra. Silently chant the four primal sounds—Saa Taa Naa Maa—directing them toward the brow.

Time. Continue for five to thirty-one minutes.[36]

Seal your practice with Sat Naam. Bring your hands together in Prayer Pose in front of your heart. Inhale deeply and either chant or say out loud "Sat Naam," which means "truth is my essence."

Affirmation

After the meditation, sit in silence and repeat the following affirmation three to five times to yourself or out loud. For extra energy, you can also write it three to five times in your journal.

> *I am not my addiction. I am releasing my addictive patterns more and more each day. I deserve happiness, peace, and healing!*

Visualization

With your eyes closed, visualize what your life will look like with this addiction healed and released. How will it change your reality? How will you feel when you wake up in the morning? Who will you be spending time with? What will you be doing? Feel what it will be like to manifest freedom from your addiction.

Nourishment

Next, hop on into the kitchen for some No-More-Cravings Millet Porridge. This hearty breakfast helps balance out any cravings and imbalances from addictions. Millet's complex carbs increase serotonin—a brain chemical known to help to improve mood and sleep—and its fiber content reduces hunger cravings.[37]

One addiction leads to another, and releasing one addiction leads to releasing another. When you balance any food cravings and release them, it will help you so much in your overall journey of leaving addictions behind, no matter what kind you are working with!

NO-MORE-CRAVINGS MILLET PORRIDGE

Prep time: 30 minutes
Makes 2 servings

1 cup millet

1 cup water

2 cups almond or coconut milk

⅛ teaspoon ground cinnamon

1 teaspoon vanilla

1 tablespoon maple syrup

Topping options: raisins, coconut flakes, berries, bananas, sliced apples, hemp seeds, maple syrup, granola, pumpkin seeds

>> In a small saucepan, combine the millet, water, milk, cinnamon, and vanilla. Bring to a boil.

Reduce the heat to low. Cover and simmer for 25 minutes without stirring. If the liquid is not completely absorbed, cook for 3 to 5 minutes longer, partially covered. Remove from the heat. Drizzle with the maple syrup and topping choices and serve!

6699

YOU HAVE AN OPPORTUNITY TO SHIFT YOUR REALITY BY COMMITTING TO THIS WORK. YOU CAN DO IT OR ELSE YOU WOULDN'T BE READING THIS. IT'S NOT ALWAYS EASY, BUT IT'S WORTH IT BECAUSE *YOU'RE* WORTH IT. DON'T STOP UNTIL YOU GET THERE! WE'RE YOUR BIGGEST CHEERLEADERS, AND WE'LL BE ROOTING FOR YOU THE WHOLE WAY THROUGH!

—XO, B+T

RITUAL 15 >>

Fountain of Youth
Feel and Look Younger

25–30 MINUTES

We're about to answer the question that has created a billion-dollar industry: How do we slow down, prevent, and reverse aging? According to yogic science, looking and feeling youthful has nothing to do with what's being promoted on Revlon commercials or in plastic surgeons' offices. Instead, it's about using your own life-force energy to slow aging from the inside out.

Kundalini yoga is full of restorative practices that allow you to not only look amazing but also to feel vibrant and have high levels of energy and vitality into your later years! These revitalizing practices are more important than ever, given that the population of people over eighty-five years old is projected to more than double from 6.4 million in 2016 to 14.6 million in 2040. (That's a 129 percent increase)![38] Clearly, we are living longer. So now, we need to figure out how to thrive and age gracefully in a world where disease is on the rise and quality of life has the potential to decline with age more than ever.

Even if you're still decades away from senior-citizen status, you can still benefit from the practices in this ritual. No matter how old you are, the choices you make at all stages of life impact how young and vibrant you feel. This is the powerful energy of the changemaker, the entrepreneur, and the "superwoman" mama or athlete! Anyone can tap into this fountain of youth and set their current and future selves up to be like one of our idols Iris Apfel, who was born in 1921 and lives her best life. (Look her up if you don't know of her!)

If we want different results than those of the average human, we need to look beyond the status quo and approach aging differently. A prematurely aging body is a body out of tune, out of shape, and most often the result of the inability to handle mental and physical stressors in its environment. This affects our quality of life in huge ways, so we are on a mission to help more people get on the vitality train! Through a lot of research and treasure hunting through the archives of yogic science (and our own experimentation), we have put together a powerful ritual that will activate more youthful energy from the inside out. So make the commitment to trade Botox for breathwork and let's get started!

Gather

- Yoga mat, meditation cushion, or chair.

- Green tourmaline crystal. This crystal is thought to open the heart chakra and keep your life-force energy flowing through your body, making it a great tool for relieving fatigue and helping with self-expression.[39] Hold your green tourmaline (or any other green crystal) between your palms with your hands in prayer position as you tune in.

- Helichrysum oil. This has actually been dubbed "the fountain of youth" because it's often used for age reversal and healing. It has anti-inflammatory, antioxidant, and antimicrobial effects, and it can help reduce stress and burnout. It's especially good for the skin with a carrier oil, like coconut oil, so use this oil in the bath with some Epsom salt to melt the stress and keep your skin looking healthy.

- Ingredients for Fountain of Youth Smoothie.

Visualization + Affirmation

Take a deep breath and powerfully exhale. Repeat the deep breaths two more times. Take a minute to sit in meditation and feel your cells vibrating.

Tap into a time in your life where you felt most alive and energized. Remember what gave you that feeling and connect it with any positive aspects of yourself that you associate with that vibrant energy. Visualize your organs being renewed, your cells invigorated, and more energy running through your chakras, your body, and your mind. Picture yourself full of zest, living life to the fullest!

Now, bring that energy into your life right now. Picture at least one thing that would be different in your day with more youthful, vibrant energy! Write it down and come back to it after the ritual to really lock it into your subconscious.

Say to yourself a few times with excited energy:

Holy shit, I'm alive! Thanks, universe, for having me back another day!

Feel free to LOL at yourself—laughing is the best youthful medicine!

Tune In

Come down onto your mat, sitting in a cross-legged position. Alternatively, you can sit in a chair with shoes off and both feet flat on the ground. Rub your palms together and bring them into your heart center in a prayer position. Begin your ritual by tuning in with the "Adi Mantra"—"Ong Namo Guroo Dayv Namo"—three times.

Mantra + Self-Care + Breathwork

We'll start by pressing play on a powerful healing mantra that will tap you into the energies of the sun, moon, earth, and infinite spirit: "Raa Maa Daa Saa Saa Say So Hung"! This one holds eight sounds that stimulate the Kundalini flow within the central channel of the spine, which will flood your system with new energy!

We love the version by Snatam Kaur, "Ra Ma da Sa (Total Healing)"—you can find it on the Spotify playlist we made to accompany this book.

Begin by rubbing a few drops of helichrysum oil and a few drops of a carrier oil, like coconut oil, in the palms of your hands and take a couple of deep breaths into your palms. Then, lightly slap your cheeks in small, upward circles giving yourself a little "wake-up" facial.

Next, you are going to do a breathing practice to stimulate the vagus nerve, which will release mood-boosting hormones, keep your mind clear, and energize your body! It releases stress and tension, which are a huge cause of illness and aging. This breathwork also activates the thyroid and parathyroid glands while increasing lung capacity.

Sit tall, pucker your lips, and whistle as you inhale. Then, exhale through the nose. If this is too difficult, you can reverse the breathing pattern so you're inhaling through the nose and exhaling through puckered lips for the whistle. Don't worry if you can't make the whistle sound—it will have the same effect if you just pucker your lips and try.

Continue this breath for two to three minutes.[40]

To end, inhale deeply through your nose, drop your shoulders away from your ears, and hold the breath for ten seconds. Exhale through your mouth, releasing all your breath.

Fun Facts About the Vagus Nerve

If you're not familiar with your vagus nerve, it's time to get acquainted! The vagus nerve is the longest nerve that extends down from the brain. It reaches all the way through your neck, chest, stomach, and colon, and has a hand in your heart rate, digestion, speech, and more. (In other words, it's kind of a big deal.)

Movement

Now, we are going to come into one of our favorite warm-ups, Frog Pose. This movement will get your cardiovascular system going, regenerate your cerebrospinal fluid, and bring energy to your life nerve, which gets tweaked and stagnant from too much sitting. (In case you were wondering, the life nerve begins in the lower back and runs through each buttock and down each leg, all the way to the back of each foot. It's different from your vagus nerve but also super important to stimulate to keep you feeling youthful.)

Stand up and then bend your knees and squat all the way down to the floor, placing your fingertips on the floor between your thighs. Now come onto your toes, pull your heels in to touch, and keep them raised off the floor, knees spread wide. Keep your head level and looking forward.

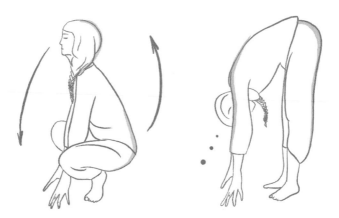

Inhale through the nose as you lift your buttocks up toward the sky, keeping your fingertips and balls of your feet on the ground. As you raise your hips, allow the top of your head to tip down toward the floor so your face is now facing your knees. Exhale through your nose as you return to the starting position.

Close your eyes and continue for twenty-six breaths, then inhale deeply into the straight-legged position with your buttocks lifted and hold your breath. Finally, exhale, come down into the squat position, and relax. Feel your cells come alive!

Meditation

Feel free to shake out your legs and grab a sip of water before we get into the meditation![41] This meditation activates the youthful energy within your body, mind, and spirit and allows you to tap into your aliveness to bring forth the special, unique qualities that only you have!

Mudra. Come into Easy Pose, with your upper arms relaxed at your sides, elbows bent, and forearms straight out from the body, parallel to the ground and each other. Your hands will be in fists with thumbs extended straight up and pulled slightly toward the body, your palms are facing each other like you're giving someone two thumbs-up!

Breath + Mantra. Inhale deeply through the nose, completely exhale and hold the breath out, and mentally chant and vibrate with the following mantra: "Saa Taa Naa Maa, Saa Taa Naa Maa, Saa Taa Naa Maa, Saa Taa Naa Maa." Then, inhale and repeat.

Eyes. Open your eyes just a bit, so you're looking through slits. They should be one-tenth open.

Time. Continue for eleven minutes.

To end. Inhale deeply and hold the breath for ten seconds. Repeat two more times and release your hands down.

Note: The Kundalini Research Institute could not verify the accuracy of these instructions.

Seal your practice with Sat Naam. Bring your hands together in Prayer Pose in front of your heart. Inhale deeply and either chant or say out loud "Sat Naam," which means "truth is my essence."

To receive the full benefits of this Kundalini yoga exercise, make sure that your fingertips are firmly contacting the mounds underneath your fingers and that your thumbs are stretched back. It may hurt, but that's only because the ego is being stretched in this meditation!

Nourishment

Although you won't reverse fine lines after one meal, it is proven that eating a healthy diet—aka real, whole, plant-based foods—will boost skin quality, improve immunity, and more. This Fountain of Youth Smoothie is antiaging and anti-inflammatory and will make you feel amazing when paired with the rest of the ritual for forty days (and beyond!). By blending up this vibrant smoothie that is loaded with vitamins, minerals, fiber, and flavor, you will assist all of this great energy work and help calm any inflammation in your body. And don't stop here: we promise that you will feel so much more lively the more fruits and veggies you eat!

FOUNTAIN OF YOUTH SMOOTHIE

Prep time: 5–10 minutes
Makes 2 small servings

2 cups baby kale

1 small beet, peeled and chopped

1 cup coconut milk or spring water

1 orange, peeled

2 cups frozen mixed berries

1 cup frozen pineapple

1 tablespoon fresh ginger, peeled and grated or chopped

1 tablespoon coconut oil

>> Place baby kale, beet, coconut milk or spring water, and orange into a blender. Puree until smooth. Add the remaining ingredients. Blend again until smooth.

Napping for eleven minutes a day is the magic amount of time according to Kundalini yoga wisdom to help your nervous system release stress, relieve fatigue in the body, and overall leave you with a sense of rejuvenation. It's one of our favorite yogic self-care tips, especially for women, that will lead to more vitality in your body.

> **"99**
>
> AGE IS JUST A NUMBER, AND WE KNOW THAT FORTY CAN BE THE NEW TWENTY. OUR FAMILY MEMBERS WHO PRACTICE THESE TECHNIQUES AND EAT HEALTHY, VEGAN FOODS LOOK TWENTY YEARS YOUNGER—AND LIVE COMPLETELY DIFFERENT LIVES—THAN OTHERS IN THEIR GENERATION. IT'S UP TO YOU TO DEFY LIMITATIONS AND LIVE THE HEALTHIEST, HAPPIEST, AND MOST ENERGIZED LIFE POSSIBLE. YOU CAN DO IT! HERE'S TO DRINKING FROM THE FOUNTAIN OF YOUTH EVERY DAY!
>
> *—XO, B+T*

RITUAL 16 >>>

Healing Heartbreak
Cut Energetic Cords to Find Your
Happiness Again

25–30 MINUTES

We can't control everything that comes our way. Crisis will inevitably arrive, and for most of us, heartbreak will be part of our life experience. When we're faced with the loss of a loved one—either because they departed this Earth or departed our lives to move on to a new path, setting us on a new path in turn—it's not easy. It can actually feel like the heartbreak physically hurts, and there's a scientific reason for that.

Neurological studies have shown that when you're "feeling hurt" after a breakup, a rejection, or a loss, it's not just a figure of speech. Physical pain and emotional pain, like heartbreak, travel along and stimulate the exact same pathways in the brain. When you feel like you have a hole in your heart after an emotional loss, this sensation is no different to your brain than if you had physically lost a limb.[42] If you're having trouble letting someone or something go, you're still connected to the relationship experience, and your body is still expecting to get a "fix" of love chemicals, like dopamine, from whomever you've lost.

Heartbreak is both an emotional and a visceral experience, and it takes energy and healing to move through it. So first, it's important to have an abundant amount of compassion for what you're going through.

When you're faced with heartbreak, you can focus on going inward and working with your soul. This process involves removing the energetic cords between you and the person you've lost, calming the heart chakra, and balancing the neurological secretions that keep you feeling the perceived pain of loss or rejection. It's also important to recognize the incredible gifts that come from heartbreak. (Yes, we're serious!) What you stand to gain through the experience is a deeper understanding of yourself. Think of it as an opportunity to dive inward on a journey of self-discovery, experiencing your incredible resilience and exploring levels of yourself that you may not have known were there.

With the right tools, you can come out on the other side of heartbreak more radiant and with an expanded view of what you're capable of handling. This is one of the reasons we love the technology of Kundalini yoga so much—there always seems to be "a meditation for that," and there actually *is* a meditation specifically for helping to heal heartbreak. (Spoiler alert: you'll do it in this ritual!)

If you're in the midst of a loss or a rejection or can't seem to move on from a situation or person, this ritual was created for you. We recommend that you commit to practicing this ritual for at least forty days to move through the portal of pain. You'll come out the other side feeling much better, with a whole new understanding of yourself.

Let's get to it, you beautiful babe. We've got you!

Gather

- Yoga mat, meditation cushion, or chair.

- Rose quartz crystal. Rose quartz is known to help to balance the emotions and heart center while raising self-esteem. Wear it as a necklace, or get a small stone and either wear it in your bra throughout the day or carry it with you in your pocket.

- Rose oil. To help alleviate the pain of heartache, deeply inhale the smell of the oil and rub a small amount on your heart center with some coconut oil before you begin this ritual.

- Ingredients for the Green Goddess Smoothie.

Tune In

Come down onto your mat, sitting in a cross-legged position. Alternatively, you can sit in a chair with shoes off and both feet flat on the ground. Rub your palms together and bring them into your heart center in a prayer position. Begin your ritual by tuning in with the "Adi Mantra"—"Ong Namo Guroo Dayv Namo"—three times.

Mantra

We'll use the mantra "Saa Taa Naa Maa"—a *bij* mantra, which acts like a seed planted in the mind—which can transform longing thoughts of your lost love to a higher vibration. It will help rewire and heal your mind and instill a sense of peace and happiness.

Saa = Infinity, Taa = Life, Naa = Death, Maa = Rebirth

Play the mantra on repeat throughout this ritual. We love the version by Mirabai Ceiba titled "Sa Ta Na Ma"—it's on the Spotify playlist we created to accompany this book!

Hit play on the "Sa Ta Na Ma" mantra and let's start healing through your heartbreak.

Play this high-vibrational mantra while you sleep to let it penetrate into your subconscious mind and accelerate your healing. The volume can be so low that you can only hear it when you put the speaker up to your ear.

Breathwork

Take a few deep belly breaths. Place your hands on your belly and inhale long and deep as you expand your belly out as far as you can. When you can't expand any further, exhale and contract your belly all the way into your spine, expelling all of your breath. As you do this, send love and appreciation for yourself through your hands and into your stomach.

Continue breathing long and deep with your hands on your belly, eyes closed, for three minutes. Then move into a short warm-up.

Warm-Up

Keep your hands on your knees and begin a heart-opening spinal flex.

Sit tall with an elongated spine and inhale as you arch your spine forward, moving from the hips and expanding your chest out. Exhale as you round out your back, contracting your spine in the opposite direction and pulling your belly in. Keep your chin parallel to the ground as you continue this movement, breathing through your nose with your eyes closed for three minutes.

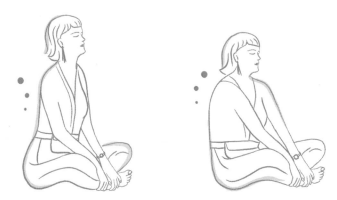

At the end of three minutes, sit tall and inhale deeply, holding the breath for a few seconds, then exhale and relax before going into the meditation.

Remember the deep belly breathing you started with? During this spinal-flex warm-up, continue expanding your stomach out as far as you can on the inhale and contracting it in as you exhale and round out your back. This technique helps to activate your lymphatic system and move toxins through the body, making you look and feel younger and more vibrant...there's more than one benefit to healing heartbreak the ETG way!

Meditation

This meditation is a Kundalini yoga technology specifically designed to heal heartbreak.[43] What you're doing in this position is stimulating the heart meridian that runs along your pinkie and outer forearm to create balance and calm the emotions felt in the heart center. This meditation steadies the pathway in the brain that stimulates that emotional and physical pain sensation—the one that tells your brain that losing a loved one feels like you've lost your arm.

Posture. Sit tall in Easy Pose or in a chair, lengthening the spine. Apply a light Neck Lock by pulling your chin down and back—you should feel a little pressure at your jawline.

Mudra. Place your palms together in front of your chest, lightly touching in a prayer position. Keeping your palms together, raise your hands up so that the tip of the Saturn (middle) finger is at the level of your third-eye point (between your eyebrows). Keep your forearms parallel to the ground and your elbows high.

Eyes. Close your eyes to look within.

Breath. Take long, deep breaths.

Time. Continue for eleven minutes.

To end. Inhale deeply, exhale fully, relax the breath, and with clasped hands, stretch the arms up overhead for two minutes. Feel your heart center and your nervous system relax a bit and fill the emptiness in your heart up with light that radiates love for yourself and for all in the situation.

Seal your practice with Sat Naam. Bring your hands together in Prayer Pose in front of your heart. Inhale deeply and either chant or say out loud "Sat Naam," which means "truth is my essence."

You can work up to doing thirty-one or sixty-two minutes of this meditation, but start with eleven to develop a relationship with it.

Visualization

Once you complete the meditation, sit in stillness listening to the "Saa Taa Naa Maa" mantra. Begin visualizing the other person involved in your heartbreak. See them standing right in front of you with a loving smile, an open heart, and kind eyes.

Begin to send them love and forgiveness. Then, send love to yourself and imagine the cord of light energy that connects you two starting to retract from the center—your energy is coming back to you and theirs is going back to them. As this happens, thank and honor them for showing up in your life in whatever capacity they did so that you could see things about yourself that you needed to see in order to grow.

Mentally say to them: "I love you. I honor you. Thank you. I set you free." Turn the focus to yourself and repeat the same affirmation "I love you. I honor you. Thank you. I set you free." Open your eyes, take a deep breath, hold it, and exhale.

Slowly get up and head to the kitchen to make a heart-healing smoothie.

Nourishment

GREEN GODDESS SMOOTHIE

Prep time: Less than 5 minutes
Makes 2 servings

1 cup pineapple or banana (preferably frozen, which will make the smoothie thicker)

½ medium avocado

2 cups spinach (packed tightly)

1 cup coconut water or coconut milk

1 teaspoon spirulina

½ teaspoon maca powder

½ teaspoon sea salt

>> In a blender, blend the spinach and coconut water or coconut milk first. Add the rest of the ingredients and blend well, until smooth. Pour and serve—that's it!

Substitution ideas: Instead of banana, try three pieces of steamed, then frozen, cauliflower. Instead of coconut, try almond milk or alkaline water. Instead of spinach, try kale.

❝❞

HEARTBREAK IS A PART OF ALL OF OUR LIVES. YOU'RE MOVING THROUGH IT WITH GRACE AND HONORING YOURSELF AND THE OTHER PARTY IN SUCH A HIGH-VIBE, COMPASSIONATE WAY. CHEERS TO YOU! KEEP IT UP, AND WE'LL SEE YOU ON THE OTHER SIDE WITH A HEART AS SOLID AS GOLD, READY TO TAKE ON YOUR NEXT LOVE ADVENTURE!

—XO, B+T

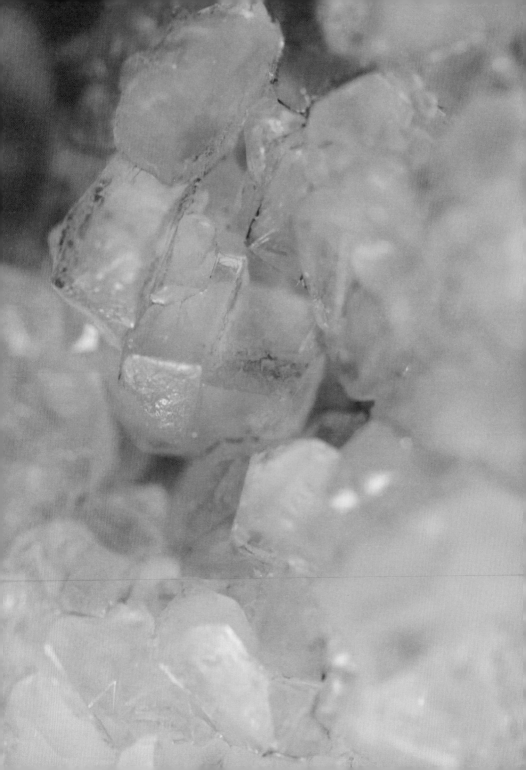

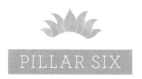

Body and Wellness

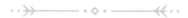

We believe it's time to approach health in a new way—one that empowers all of us to feel physically strong and gives us the vitality to do amazing things in the world with a high quality of life. To us, this means striving to live preventively and taking care of our bodies versus reactively treating sickness once it's already here. That's why wellness is a huge part of our lifestyle. After all, if our "meat suits" aren't working for us here in this human experience, then nothing else matters.

With the help of Kundalini yoga, lots of veggies, plenty of long walks, and a little law-of-attraction magic, we're setting ourselves up to have the best possible chance of cat-cowing as long as we both shall live! (On our long-term vision boards, you better believe we're ninety-five, teaching yoga, and doing high kicks.)

According to Kundalini wisdom, vibrant health starts by nourishing the main systems of the body: the immune system, nervous system, and endocrine system. Then, we work with our masculine and feminine energies to make sure that our chakras, hormones, and minds are balanced. We also look at how we are using our bodies to operate in the world—either in a balanced way that flows with nature or an imbalanced way that feeds into aging and disease. (All while making sure that the relationship with our bodies is positive and loving in the process!) When we create practices that nurture these systems of our body, we are able to help them function at their highest capacity. This gives us the best chance at overall wellness and high levels of functioning—get ready to take your body and wellness to another level of greatness!

Immune Upgrade
Immune System

25-30 MINUTES

You might not think about your immune system unless you're sick, but this built-in defense mechanism works hard for you every day. In today's society, we are exposed to so many toxins—from environmental pollution to pesticides in food and chemicals in household products. The amazing thing is when your immune system is strong and vital, it is always adapting to your environment to keep you strong.

Boosting your immune system isn't just about getting your vitamin C. The thoughts and feelings you entertain on a daily basis play a big part in how well your immune system can protect your body against illness.[44] That's why it's so important to have daily practices to preventively boost and strengthen it!

According to Kundalini yoga, the lymphatic system, the glandular system, and the aura all play a role in our overall immunity. In this ritual, we work with a variety of tools to boost these systems: crystals, mantra, breathwork, meditation, and movement. We're all about giving ourselves the best chance to stay healthy and well so we can show up in the world feeling our best as much as humanly possible. (As we've figured out by using these amazing energy and mind-set tools, that can actually be a lot of the time!)

Gather

- Yoga mat, meditation cushion, or chair.

- Amber crystal. A powerful healer and purifier, amber strengthens vitality while absorbing pain, negativity, and stress.

- Ingredients for Immune-Boosting Morning Shot.

Movement

We'll start with warming up the body with some yogic jumping jacks! Begin in a standing position and jump your feet out to the sides as you clap your palms above your head. Then, as you jump your feet together, slap your hands on the sides of your thighs. Do ten of these.

Now, slowly come down to sitting in Easy Pose for one more warm-up before we get into our breathwork and meditation.

Bring your hands into Prayer Pose at the center of your chest, then extend your arms out to the sides, and then return them to Prayer Pose. Continue, stretching the armpits as much as you can when you extend the arms out to the sides. Breathe long and deep. Keep moving faster and faster, extending the arms all the way out. You are exercising your immune system and making it stronger.

After three minutes, start getting angry and feisty. Use the motion to get all your anger out. Continue for another five to eight minutes and really move any stagnant, low-vibrational energy that is weighing you down!

Tune In

Sitting in your cross-legged position, or alternatively, sitting in a chair with shoes off and both feet flat on the ground, rub your palms together and bring them into your heart center in a prayer position. Begin your ritual by tuning in with the "Adi Mantra"—"Ong Namo Guroo Dayv Namo"—three times.

Bring the amber crystal into your hands and tap into your intuition, holding it on any part of your body that needs a little extra love and healing. Then, feel free to place it in front of you for the rest of the ritual.

Breathwork + Mantra

Now, we are going to go into some breathwork that brings energy to your immune system.[45] It's a very healing exercise that is especially great to do if you are fighting an infection. You may start to feel tingling in your toes, thighs, and lower back after a bit—that is an indication that you are doing this exercise correctly, so don't worry if it feels weird! It's just the energy moving and upgrading.

Feel free to play the mantra "Raa Maa Daa Saa, Saa Say So Hung" during this part of the ritual. (We love the version on our Spotify playlist by White Sun!) This is an extremely healing mantra that will uplift your vibration and your immune system through the sacred sound currents.

To start the breathwork, stay sitting in Easy Pose with your chin in and your chest out. Stick your tongue all the way out and keep it out as you rapidly breathe in and out through your mouth like a dog panting (aka dog breath). As you inhale, your stomach comes out, and as you exhale, it will contract in. Continue this panting diaphragmatic breath for three to five minutes.

To finish, inhale, and hold your breath for fifteen seconds while pressing the tongue against the upper palate. Exhale and relax.

Meditation

We are now going to hop, skip, and jump into the immune system booster: the Inner Sun Meditation. This is an advanced immune therapy that is said to release viruses and bacteria while strengthening the system! The feelings of anger, self-defeat, and blame block the flow of our inner strength, and to boost the immune system we have to bust through these blocks. That's what this meditation is designed to do—prepare to get a little emotional! Lightness, hope, and energy are on the other side.

For this one, the head must be covered with a beanie, hat, scarf, headband, or turban—otherwise, you could get a headache.

Posture. Sit in Easy Pose, with a light neck lock (called Jalandhar Bandh), and with the head covered. To create a neck lock, tuck in your chin so your neck is totally straight. Chest is out. Feel the stretch across the chest.

Mudra. Bend the left arm and raise the hand up to shoulder level. The palm faces forward. The forearm is perpendicular to the ground. Make Surya Mudra with the left hand (touch the tip of the ring finger to the tip of the thumb). The mudra of the left hand may slip during practice; keep it steady. Make a fist of the right hand, pressing the tips of the fingers into the pads at the base of the fingers; extend the index finger. With the extended index finger, gently close off the right nostril.

Focus. Concentrate at the brow point.

Breath. Begin a steady, powerful Breath of Fire. Emphasize the breath at the navel; the navel must move. Note: If you're on the first three days of your moon cycle or you're pregnant, do long, deep breathing instead.

Mantra. Though this is done without a mantra, you may want to use a mantra recording for the proper rhythm. A good recording for the rhythm is Sada Sat Kaur's "Angel's Waltz," which we've included within the Spotify playlist that accompanies this book.

Time. Continue for three minutes. Very gradually increase the time to five minutes and up to thirty-one minutes.

To end. Inhale deeply and hold the breath. As you hold the breath, interlace all the fingers (beginning with the right thumb on top) and put the palms in front just below the throat and about fourteen inches away from the body. Try to pull the fingers apart with all your force. Resist and create a great tension. When you must, exhale. Repeat this sequence three more times. On the last exhale, discharge the breath by blowing through your upturned lips, with the tongue curled back on the roof of the mouth. This will seal the upper palate upward. Then relax.

Seal your practice with Sat Naam. Bring your hands together in Prayer Pose in front of your heart. Inhale deeply and either chant or say out loud "Sat Naam," which means "truth is my essence."

Affirmation

After the meditation, sit in silence and repeat the following affirmation three to five times to yourself or out loud. For extra energy, you can also write it three to five times in your journal.

I am strong and protected in all ways! My immune system and all systems of my body are working for me, and I am becoming healthier every day!

Visualization

Picture your body and all of your systems working to their highest capacity. Visualize any sickness or ailments completely healed and see yourself in a perfectly healthy, vital state!

Nourishment

After your visualization, pour yourself a shot!! An Immune-Boosting Morning Shot, that is. It'll be better than a cup of coffee and the perfect complement to all of this amazing work you just did!

IMMUNE-BOOSTING MORNING SHOT

Prep time: 5 minutes
Makes 1 cup

- 1–2 cloves garlic
- 1 tablespoon maple syrup (optional)
- ¼ teaspoon turmeric powder
- 1 tablespoon hot water
- Juice of 1 lemon
- Juice of 1 navel orange
- 1 teaspoon fresh ginger, peeled and grated
- Dash of cayenne pepper
- Dash of sea salt
- Grind of black pepper
- 1 tablespoon apple cider vinegar with "the Mother"

>> Mince the garlic (ideally put through a garlic press) and set aside for 10 minutes. (This gives the enzymes a chance to form and ensures maximum benefits.) Whisk together the maple syrup, turmeric, and hot water until every-thing is incorporated and smooth. Stir in everything else including the garlic, and shoot it down!

You can make enough for the week and put it in an airtight container. Then, all you have to do is pour it every day!

> ❝❞
>
> YOU OWE IT TO YOURSELF TO HEAL ANYTHING THAT IS
> PREVENTING YOU FROM EXPERIENCING LIFE FULLY! IT MAY
> FEEL LIKE A LOT OF EFFORT OR EVEN DIFFICULT AT TIMES
> ALONG THE JOURNEY, BUT THERE IS NOTHING MORE
> IMPORTANT YOU CAN PUT YOUR TIME OR ENERGY INTO.
> KEEP IT UP, AND YOUR WHOLE WORLD WILL START TO
> GET A LOT BRIGHTER. BRING ON THE SUN!
>
> *—XO, B+T*

Energy Boost
Nervous System

20-30 MINUTES

Energy is our greatest human currency. Nothing else holds more weight. Having more energy equals higher-vibe emotions, better health and vitality, and the ability to easily attract love, health, and abundance in all forms.

Are you in need of an energy boost? Maybe you've got the obvious signs—feeling lethargic throughout the day or having trouble taking action on the things you want to get done. Or perhaps your symptoms are more subtle: when we're tired, we often feel a heaviness and tend to resort to habits that we're trying to transform, like that extra cup of coffee, a sugary snack, or skipping a workout to binge-watch Netflix because we just can't imagine having to get off the couch.

Instead of borrowing energy from things outside of yourself, you can use yogic techniques to tap into the infinite amount of energy available to you always. These tools will give you more energy simply by moving your body or taking in more *pranic* life-force energy (aka more breath).

This ritual is designed to give you a daily energy boost while upgrading your nervous system to be able to handle more as you create more in your life. The more you practice these tools, the more energy you will cultivate. Both the breathwork technique and the meditation are tools you can use at any point through your day to give you that get-up-and-go you're reaching for.

Gather

- Yoga mat, meditation cushion, or chair.

- Citrine crystal. Citrine radiates positivity, joy, and a lot of energy! Place it in your meditation space while you do this ritual, or to enhance its qualities and work with your energy all day, wear it around your neck on a long chain so it hits your diaphragm where your willpower resides. You can also wear it on either of your ring fingers, which are both connected to that blazing energy source in our universe, the sun.

- Saffron, orange, and frankincense oils. These essential oils are connected to the sun and can help relax a frazzled nervous system. Add any of these oils to a carrier oil such as almond oil and place a drop or two in your palms, rub your hands together, and cover your face with your hands. Take three deep inhales before you begin this ritual.

- Ingredients for Good Morning Matcha Smoothie.

Tune In

Come down onto your mat, sitting in a cross-legged position. Alternatively, you can sit in a chair with shoes off and both feet flat on the ground. Rub your palms together and bring them into your heart center in a prayer position. Begin your ritual by tuning in with the "Adi Mantra"—"Ong Namo Guroo Dayv Namo"—three times.

Mantra

Press play on the "Aadee Shaktee" mantra, which calls upon the universal Divine Mother energy. This mantra taps into the primal creative force to raise your Kundalini energy and help you manifest your desires. We love the version by Sada Sat Kaur called "Adi Shakti." You can find it on the Spotify playlist we made to accompany this book!

Breathwork

You're going to practice an energizing breath that connects you to the sun's energy, which gives you a boost of power to get through your day.[46] Sitting with a tall spine in Easy Pose—a seated cross-legged position—block your left nostril with the thumb of your left hand, keeping the other four fingers straight up, like antennae connecting you to the sun. Take twenty-six slow, long, deep, and complete breaths through your right nostril only. After you complete twenty-six breaths, unblock your left nostril, inhale deeply, and relax.

Our right nostril is connected to the sun, and our left nostril to the moon, so by breathing through your right nostril only, you're recharging yourself and generating heat, power, and vitality.

Warm-Up

We'll start moving our body with Bundle Rolls. You may feel like a child playing while you're doing this movement! It's super fun and surprisingly invigorating, and the bonus is that it feels like a full body massage. Begin by lying on your back and pulling your arms tight against the sides of your body. Extend your legs out in front of you and squeeze them together. Use your core to lift your legs, neck, and shoulders a couple inches off the ground, keeping your arms locked to your sides and legs squeezed together. Using your pelvis, thrust your body over to the right side and then roll back to the left side. Keep going back and forth to each side. You will look and feel like a rolling log, and the more momentum you create, the easier it will be to sustain the motion. Go at a pace that feels good for you for two to three minutes.

Meditation

Come back into Easy Pose to give yourself a jump start with this meditation, which will start to energize your own electromagnetic field.[47] It's a great way to start your morning or to use as a pick-me-up throughout the day.

Posture. Sit in Easy Pose with your hands in Gyan Mudra (index fingertips and thumb tips touch). Like an old-fashioned eggbeater, rotate your hands around each other, over and over in front of your heart center. Move very quickly (about six circles per second). If your hands get tangled, just start again.

Eyes. Eyes are one-tenth open, so you can see a little sliver of light coming through your eyelids.

Breath. Take long, deep breaths through the nose.

Time. Continue this movement for three minutes. You can work up to eleven minutes with practice.

To end. Fully close your eyes, inhale deeply, and lift your arms straight up to the sky with no bend in your elbows. Breathe long and deep here for one more minute, stretching your arms up as far as you can, then relax your arms down to your knees.

Seal your practice with Sat Naam. Bring your hands together in Prayer Pose in front of your heart. Inhale deeply and either chant or say out loud "Sat Naam," which means "truth is my essence."

Visualization

Sitting in silence with your hands on your knees, take a moment to scan your body and feel the difference in your cells and in the energy you feel directly around you. Visualize a bright, yellow light burning bright like the sun at your navel. Watch this bright sun energy charge up your navel point as it gets brighter and brighter, beginning to encompass your whole body and charge every cell. You're now bathing in this bright yellow energizing and invigorating light. Sit in this energy for as long as you need to.

Self-Care

Low energy is often a result of needing to increase physical activity. Make it a goal to get in more exercise throughout your days, especially while practicing this ritual. You can do this by scheduling workouts on your calendar each week to create more structure for yourself or commit to getting five thousand steps in each day by either walking or running. There are many apps that can track this for you.

If you work in an office, consider asking your coworkers to take your meetings outside on a walk. Try meeting up with friends to go to a yoga or workout class. It's important, especially for women, to sweat at least fifteen minutes a day to keep the body and mind youthful and full of vitality.

Nourishment

This stimulating smoothie will take your energy-boosting ritual to another level! Reach for it in the morning or as your 3:00 p.m. pick-me-up instead of the coffee or sugary treat that will leave you with a low-energy hangover. While matcha still contains caffeine, the phytonutrient L-theanine allows the caffeine to be absorbed at a slower rate than coffee, helping you avoid a crash.

GOOD MORNING MATCHA SMOOTHIE

Prep time: 5 minutes
Makes 1 large or 2 small servings
(keep some later for an afternoon snack!)

Handful of spinach or kale

1 small banana, peeled

1 orange, peeled

1 teaspoon matcha tea powder

1 cup almond milk (or any plant-based milk)

>> Put all of your ingredients in the blender and blend until smooth! Enjoy!

YOU ARE BURSTING WITH LIGHT, YOU BEAUTIFUL LIGHTBEING! SPREAD YOUR LOVE TO EVERYONE YOU MEET TODAY! YOU NOW HAVE ENOUGH ENERGY TO ACCOMPLISH EVERYTHING THAT NEEDS TO GET DONE—THE UNIVERSE IS WORKING FOR YOU, AND ALL YOU HAVE TO DO IS SHOW UP.

—XO, B+T

Balanced Hormones
Endocrine System

30-35 MINUTES

A healthy and balanced endocrine system makes for a healthy body and mind. When any part of this system is out of whack, it can feel like everything in your body is off-balance, including your appetite, weight, mood, and sex drive. The endocrine system is ruled by the master of all glands—the pituitary gland—and is made up of a complex network of glands that includes the hypothalamus, pineal gland, thyroid, parathyroid, thymus, adrenals, pancreas, ovaries, and testes. All of these glands produce various hormones that control a number of vital organs in the body, so it's important that they all work together and at their best capacity.

In yogic philosophy, the glands are considered to be the "guardians of health" because of how important they are in keeping harmony within the body. Stimulating, adjusting, and refreshing this system can do wonders for our overall health and balance.

The endocrine system is quite intricate, so instead of pinpointing just one gland to balance out, we can go right to the pituitary "master gland," located in the brain behind the bridge of the nose. The pituitary gland works with the hypothalamus, which connects to the nervous system and relays information back to the pituitary on how much of each hormone the glands need to produce. It's the command center for hormones!

In this ritual, we will march directly to that hormone command post and revitalize the pituitary gland as a means to refresh and reset the endocrine system.

Bonus: Your intuition may also get a boost, because the pituitary gland is connected to the third-eye chakra—the energy center responsible for our intuition, vision, and clarity on where we are going in life! Let's get to it!

Gather

- Yoga mat, meditation cushion, or chair.

- Moonstone crystal. Moonstone is connected to the moon, which affects the tides of the ocean. Similarly, it's thought to calm turbulent emotions by helping balance hormones in the body. Hold the moonstone during the visualization potion of the ritual and/or wear moonstone as jewelry throughout the day.

- Clary sage oil. Rub a couple drops on your abs, inside your forearms, and/or behind your ears before you begin this ritual. If you're sensitive to essential oils, use a carrier oil like coconut oil to dilute. Clary sage is great for women specifically because it helps to reduce stress hormone levels and relax the body. Place a couple of drops in your diffuser prior to beginning your ritual (please do not use if you're pregnant). [48]

- Fruit, greens, and ashwagandha powder for your breakfast.

Tune In

Come down onto your mat, sitting in a cross-legged position. Alternatively, you can sit in a chair with shoes off and both feet flat on the ground. Rub your palms together and bring them into your heart center in a prayer position. Begin your ritual by tuning in with the "Adi Mantra"—"Ong Namo Guroo Dayv Namo"—three times.

Mantra

Press play on the mantra we'll use for this entire ritual: "Whaa-hay Guroo." The essence of this mantra expresses the indescribable experience of moving from ignorance to understanding through experience and knowledge. It also triggers destiny in you, and because we're working with the pituitary gland and our third eye, we may just start to see the pathway! We love "Tantric Wahe Guru" by Snatam Kaur on her album *Meditations for Transformation 1: Merge & Flow*. You can find it on the Spotify playlist we've made to accompany this book!

Warm-Up

Remain sitting in Easy Pose and place your hands on your knees. Begin to slowly circle your head to the right. Focus on warming up the neck and moving as slowly as you need to. Close your eyes. Breathe long and deep through your nose wwas you make full circles with your head. Continue this movement for two minutes in each direction. This will begin to wake up an important part of the endocrine system—your thyroid.

After you've completed two minutes on each side, bring your neck to a neutral position. Inhale deeply and relax, dropping your shoulders away from your ears.

Begin to chant "Wahe Guru" along with the mantra you're listening to. You are creating a sound current that has a powerful stimulating effect on the glands in your body, helping to bring your endocrine system into balance. Keep your eyes closed and get lost in chanting for three minutes. If you don't have the musical version of the mantra available, you can chant "Whaa-hay Guroo" continually in a monotone voice.

Meditation

Next, we'll move into a three-part meditation called the Sneezing Buddha Kriya.[49] The first posture will begin to stimulate the pituitary gland, and it's kind of fun (and funny!) to practice. You'll start to feel the energy around a vertical valve in your throat as you breathe this way—this valve is connected directly to the pituitary gland and invokes it throughout the meditation.

PART 1

Posture. Sit in Easy Pose with your spine straight, pulling your chin down and back so your spine feels tall and you feel a little pressure in your throat. Rest your hands in your lap any way that's comfortable.

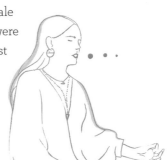

Breath. Inhale deeply through an O-shaped mouth as if you were powerfully sucking air through a straw. Then close your mouth and exhale powerfully through both nostrils as if you were sneezing the breath out. The exhale should be fast and powerful, similar to when you actually sneeze.

Eyes. Keep your eyes closed throughout the meditation.

Time. Continue this breath pattern for three minutes.

To end. Inhale deeply through your mouth, exhale through your nose, and relax, keeping your hands in your lap.

PART 2

Posture. Bend your elbows and lift them away from the body, bringing the hands about shoulder height, fingers lightly spread, palms facing upward. Your hands may become heavy during this part.

Breath. Begin breathing rapidly in and out through an O-shaped mouth using your navel point (the energy center located two to three inches below the belly button) and your diaphragm to power your breath. Make it a consistent breath and create a quick rhythm. You are cleansing the lungs, giving the blood massive amounts of oxygen and taking away disease. If you're pregnant or on the first three days of your moon cycle, do long, deep breathing.

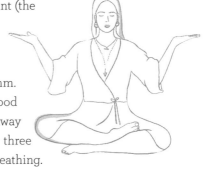

Eyes. Keep your eyes closed throughout the meditation.

Time. Continue this breath pattern for three minutes. Then immediately go into part 3.

PART 3

Posture. Now stretch your arms out to the sides, parallel to the floor; elbows are straight. Your right palm faces up toward the Heavens, and the left hand faces down toward the Earth.

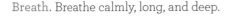

Breath. Breathe calmly, long, and deep.

Eyes. Keep your eyes closed throughout the meditation.

You are now balancing Heaven and Earth. Meditate on this balance. Within about a minute and a half, you may start to freak out because this exercise puts pressure on the pituitary gland. Just stay calm and continue to breathe long and deep. Train your brain that you are not going to give up no matter what. If you need to come out of the posture, that's okay, just use your intuition about when to come back into the posture to finish.

Time. Continue for five minutes.

To end. Hold this position and begin Breath of Fire for fifteen seconds, where you inhale and exhale, equal in strength and length, through the nose. Allow the navel point to move with the breath, expanding on the inhale, contracting on the exhale. If you're pregnant or on the first three days of your moon cycle, do long, deep breathing.

Then inhale, interlock your hands, and stretch them overhead while holding your breath for ten seconds. Stretch your spine up, exhale, and repeat this movement two more times.

Seal your practice with Sat Naam. Bring your hands together in Prayer Pose in front of your heart. Inhale deeply and either chant or say out loud "Sat Naam," which means "truth is my essence."

Visualization

Sit here, or lie on your back, and continue to listen to the "Whaa-hay Guroo" mantra, or rest in silence for three to five minutes. Focus your energy on your pituitary gland right behind the bridge of your nose. Visualize a waterfall of bright, white, light energy moving from your pituitary gland down into your throat, refreshing your thyroid; then down into the middle of your upper chest, washing over your thymus; moving further down into your lower ribs energizing your adrenal glands and pancreas; and continuing down into your ovaries or testes, washing them in this bright, refreshing light. Feel all of your glands coming online to your awareness.

Affirmation

Repeat this affirmation three times:

My body is refreshed, my glands are strong, my hormones are regulated, and I am energized!

Open your eyes and take a moment to celebrate what you just did for your mind and body. Know that every day you are moving your body and mind into a more harmonious vibration.

Self Care + Nourishment

When your body is out of balance in any way, you can help reestablish harmony through the food you consume as fuel. Like the old saying says, "You are what you eat." Try adding more fruits and greens to every meal—yes, even greens like spinach and kale for breakfast!—and reduce the amount of processed foods you consume. These foods typically have high amounts of sugar, which can be taxing on the body to process. The more whole and colorful foods you can eat, the more balance you will create in the body...so taste the rainbow!

For even more endocrine-balancing power, you can add a supplement called ashwagandha to your breakfast. The Ayurvedic tradition has been using ashwagandha for over three thousand years to support thyroid, adrenal, and reproductive hormones—among many others! It's an apoptogenic herb native to India and North Africa that helps balance the endocrine system at a cellular level, aiding you in the energetic work you've just done in this ritual.[50] It's commonly found in powder form and can be added to your morning smoothie, oatmeal bowl, plant-protein shake, or anything else that you can sneak it in!

> **❝❞**
>
> CONGRATS, BABE! THE WORK YOU'RE DOING IS CHANGING YOUR MIND, BODY, AND EMOTIONS. THIS IS SO IMPORTANT FOR YOUR OVERALL HEALTH AND WELL-BEING! **GO OUT THERE TODAY AND SHINE,** KNOWING YOU'RE CREATING BALANCE AND HARMONY WITHIN, AND YOUR WORLD WILL BEGIN TO REFLECT THAT BACK TO YOU!
>
> *—XO, B+T*

RITUAL 20 >>

Feminine Support
Pregnancy, Postpartum, Menstrual Cycle

35 MINUTES

No matter what gender you identify with, it's important to look at the balance of feminine and masculine energy within yourself and to use both of these energies in your daily life. The divine feminine is the awakened creative force that brings all things into existence. Embodying this essence brings forth a warrior spirit and the intuition and awareness to elevate your own life and serve the greater good. Feminine energy nurtures ideas into full creations, and it can be channeled in all sorts of ways: from painting, cooking, and poetry to birthing children, leading corporations, creating massive change on the planet, or all of the above. Plus, it's all about having a strong connection to emotions and feelings in the process!

If you are operating too much from your masculine energy—which is analytical, action-oriented, and all about hunting, pursuing, and chasing—you may have trouble stepping into the more feminine roles of wife and mother. It may also be more difficult for you to manifest from your soul in the way you want. But don't worry—tapping deeper into your feminine energy is a beautiful opportunity to shift versus a problem that needs to be fixed. After all, that's the feminine mind-set to get you to where you want to be!

Since our feminine energy affects all parts of our lives and our future manifestations, we created this ritual to help you boost that feminine energy no matter what you're seeking to create. Each element of this practice will bring more *shakti*—empowered feminine energy—into your life to balance the masculine, which is a powerful way to heal yourself and the planet! It's also very beneficial for people who want to get pregnant, are already pregnant or postpartum, or need menstrual cycle support. Practice it every day for forty days, and this ritual will augment your intention to fully reawaken the qualities of the sacred feminine and embody the goddess within! Get ready to feel sexy, empowered, and beautiful, because that is what you are!

Gather

- Yoga mat, meditation cushion, or chair.

- Moonstone crystal. Moonstone is the perfect crystal for tapping into lunar, feminine, yin energy! It helps you connect to your intuition and create a space of shakti flow, peace, and harmony within. We suggest placing the moonstone in your bra or pocket, keeping it close to your body during your practice, or wearing moonstone jewelry as a reminder to channel the feminine energy within you all day long.

- Jasmine oil. Jasmine has been nicknamed as the "queen of the night" (YES, please!) for its beautiful, seductive fragrance. It's perfect for the self-care portion of this ritual, and you can also use it in baths or any other time you feel called.

- Ingredients for Divine Feminine Hibiscus Rose Latte.

Warm-Up

To begin, let's warm up your body. Come down onto your mat on your hands and knees with your wrists directly under your shoulders and your palms spread wide, pressing into the ground. Feel free to place a blanket under your knees if you need some extra cushioning. Bring your knees a little bit wider than hip-width—if you are pregnant, bring them as wide as needed to create space for your baby and the movement—and start to circle your hips to the right. You can either make smaller circles just around the navel point (the energy center located two to three inches below the belly button) or larger circles, bringing your hips all the way down to your heels with each circle; do whatever feels best. Inhale through your nose as your hips come forward and exhale through the mouth as they circle around to the back.

Do this for one to three minutes, then switch directions with your circles and go to the opposite side for one to three minutes.

When you are done, come back to center with a neutral, flat spine. Take a deep inhale and exhale.

Feel free to stand up at this point in the ritual, put on your favorite song or mantra, and intuitively move your body however you want to. Dancing is a powerful way to bring in this goddess energy throughout your day—maybe even try out an ecstatic dance event or dance class!

Tune In

Make your way back to Easy Pose, sitting in a cross-legged position on your mat. Alternatively, you can sit in a chair with shoes off and both feet flat on the ground. Rub your palms together and bring them into your heart center in a prayer position. Begin your ritual by tuning in with the "Adi Mantra"—"Ong Namo Guroo Dayv Namo"—three times.

Breathwork + Mantra

To start, we will practice sitting in silence with some breathwork and mantra. Just *being* without doing is a very feminine act. If it feels difficult at first, just allow yourself to feel what comes up. Use the breath and mantra to clear any resistant energy that wants to always be on the masculine go, go, go!

Place your hands on your heart or your yoni (female organs) with your thumb tips touching and your index fingers touching, creating a triangle. Start to practice long, deep breathing—inhale through your nose and expand your stomach out, then exhale through your nose, gently contracting your stomach in. Focus on this magical life-force energy going in and out of your body temple and move into a rhythmic flow with your breath.

On the inhale, mentally say, "I am." Then, on the exhale, say, "I am a goddess of love." (You can also use any other "I am" statement that makes you feel the feminine energy awaken inside.)

Continue for one to three minutes.

Meditation + Mantra

Feel free to shake out your legs and massage them to help with circulation. Then, bring your legs back into Easy Pose for the very powerful Kundalini meditation to call upon the divine feminine energy. This meditation, called Maha Shakti, invokes divine protection, feminine flow, and energy to fulfill your desires and bring in abundance.[51] It's highly beneficial and recommended during pregnancy but can be done at any time!

Before you begin, press play on the "Aadee Shaktee" mantra—you will chant this during the meditation. There are many recorded versions of this mantra by artists such as Dev Suroop Kaur, Nirinjan Kaur, and Snatam Kaur, and you can find them on our Spotify playlist. When you chant and vibrate the "Aadee Shaktee" mantra, it is an act of devotion that aligns you to the creative feminine power of the universe.

Aadee Shaktee

Aadee Shaktee, Aadee Shakti, Aadee Shaktee, Namo Namo

Sarab Shaktee, Sarab Shaktee, Sarab Shaktee, Namo Namo

Pritham Bhagvatee, Pritham Bhagvatee, Pritham Bhagvatee Namo Namo

Kundalinee Maat Shaktee, Maat Shaktee, Namo Namo

Posture. Sit peacefully in Easy Pose with a straight spine. Make fists with your hands with both index fingers stretched out and pointing straight up. Elbows are bent and relaxed by your sides.

Mantra. As you chant the "Aadee Shaktee" mantra, hear the vibration as a vast, cosmic flow of the Divine Mother. Merge in it. This is enough to take away your misfortune, to let prosperity in, and allow your feminine power to come through you.

Eyes. Eyes are closed.

Time. Continue for eleven minutes. You can work up to thirty-one minutes.

To end. Take a deep breath in and hold. Exhale and meditate within.

Seal your practice with Sat Naam. Bring your hands together in Prayer Pose in front of your heart. Inhale deeply and either chant or say out loud "Sat Naam," which means "truth is my essence."

Within the Kundalini Yoga tradition, it is practiced that 120 days after conception the child's soul enters into the womb of its mother. This is a day of celebration when it's traditional to chant the "Aadee Shaktee" mantra—we highly recommend doing this meditation on that day when you're pregnant!

Self-Care

Place a few drops of jasmine oil in a carrier oil, such as coconut or almond oil. Bring your hands to your nose and breathe in the fragrance of the oil, and then give yourself a little foot or neck massage!

Affirmation

After this ritual or throughout your day, feel free to say these affirmations three to five times, three to five times a day!

I embrace my most powerful, expansive, complex, sexy, wild-woman self.

I welcome all aspects of my feminine, even those parts of myself that I have previously shamed or kept in the shadows.

I release the fears that keep me from expressing all of the dimensions of me as woman.

Nourishment

Finally, head to the kitchen to make our Divine Feminine Hibiscus Rose Latte. This tonic is calming, stress reducing, and the perfect warming start to your day!

DIVINE FEMININE HIBISCUS ROSE LATTE

Prep time: 10 minutes
Makes 1 serving

- 1 cup coconut milk
- 1 hibiscus tea bag or leaves
- 2 teaspoons rose water
- 1 teaspoon vanilla extract
- 1 heaping teaspoon coconut oil
- 1 teaspoon maple syrup (optional)
- 1 teaspoon rose petals

>> Bring the coconut milk to a boil in a pan on the stove and then steep the hibiscus tea in the coconut milk. Remove and discard hibiscus. Blend with the rest of the ingredients except the rose petals in a blender or with a frother and sprinkle the rose petals on top. Et voilà—a goddess drink to start the day!

66 99

YOU GO, GODDESS! **YOU ARE WAKING UP THE DIVINE FEMININE ENERGY WITHIN AND NO MATTER WHAT STAGE OR PHASE OF YOUR LIFE YOU ARE IN,** YOU ARE DOING THIS FOR YOU. WE ARE SO PROUD OF YOU! NOW DANCE YOUR WAY INTO THE FLOW OF YOUR DAY AND KNOW THAT YOU ARE BLISSFUL AND BEAUTIFUL, AND ALL OF YOUR DESIRES ARE FLOWING TO YOU ALWAYS!

—XO B+T

RITUAL 21 >>

Masculine Support
*Increase Willpower and
Self-Discipline*

25-30 MINUTES

We all have both masculine and feminine energy within us, no matter which gender we identify with. It's important to balance these two polarities within our physical bodies for our mental, physical, and spiritual health. Masculine energy is often equated with being aggressive, competitive, and controlling, but that's its wounded or weak version. In this ritual, we're cultivating divine masculine energy—a spirit of presence, focus, stability, humility, and protection. When in balance, masculine energy dances in time with the divine feminine energy within us, which is intuitive, grounded, receptive, compassionate, and trusting. (If you find that you need to support your feminine energy as well, see the "Feminine Support" ritual in this book!)

So how do you know whether your masculine energy needs to be a little stronger? If you need a boost in self-confidence, critical thinking, self-discipline, or assertiveness—or if you want to dial up or balance out your sex drive—this ritual is designed for you. It will help you connect to the divine masculine energy within you that's strong and calm, knows when to take action, and has enough energetic space to make clear decisions on how to move forward. And, yes, women can practice this ritual too—commit to it for forty days and watch your willpower, mental discipline, and courage soar!

Gather

- Yoga mat, meditation cushion, or chair.

- Citrine crystal. Keep this energizing crystal nearby on your mat as a support tool. When you go into relaxation, place it on your belly button to support your solar plexus, which is the seat of willpower in your body.

- Sandalwood oil. Place one or two drops of the oil mixed with a carrier oil like coconut oil into your palms, and rub it around your belly button to increase the energy in your solar plexus.

- Ingredients for Sun God Shatavari Smoothie.

Tune In

Come down onto your mat, sitting in a cross-legged position. Alternatively, you can sit in a chair with shoes off and both feet flat on the ground. Rub your palms together and bring them into your heart center in a prayer position. Begin your ritual by tuning in with the "Adi Mantra"—"Ong Namo Guroo Dayv Namo"—three times.

Mantra

Press play on the mantra "Har Singh Nar Singh," which helps to clear negative feelings toward the male gender and connects you directly to the divine masculine force within you. We love the version on Nirinjan Kaur's album *Adhara* titled "Har Singh Nar Singh." You can find it on the Spotify playlist we made to accompany this book!

Sit and meditate on this mantra silently for one minute and feel the mantra move through your body. Then, begin chanting along with the mantra for another two minutes. (You can hum along until you know the words.) When complete, deeply inhale, exhale, and come up to standing. You can allow the music to continue playing on repeat.

Warm-Up

We'll begin with Archer Pose, which builds physical stamina, willpower, and courage.[52]

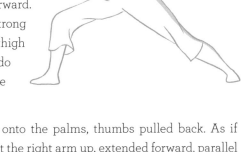

Posture. Bring the right foot forward so that the feet are two to three feet apart. The right toes face forward while the left foot comes to a forty-five-degree angle, with the heel back and the toes forward. The left leg stays straight and strong as the right knee bends until the thigh is almost parallel to the ground (do not let the knee go beyond the toes); tuck the tailbone.

Curl the fingers of both hands onto the palms, thumbs pulled back. As if pulling back a bow and arrow, lift the right arm up, extended forward, parallel to the ground, over the right knee. The left arm, bent at the elbow, pulls back until the fist is at the left shoulder.

Pull Neck Lock by tucking your chin in so your neck is totally straight. Chest is out and feel this stretch across the chest.

Eyes. Eyes stare beyond the thumb to infinity.

Breath. Make your breath long and deep through the nose.

Time. Practice for three minutes on each side.

Once you've moved through these six beautiful minutes, come back down onto your mat and get ready to practice a fundamental Kundalini yoga exercise that massages all of your internal organs. If done daily, it keeps your body clean like a temple of worship. The rhythmic motion of energy circulates through the body, energizing it and healing imbalances—especially those related to the sex organs and lower chakras—all in just a few minutes. You're starting your day with a yogic power move.

Meditation

If the mantra "Har Singh Nar Singh" is still playing, hit pause because we're going to be chanting during this meditation, which is called Sat Kriya.

Come to sitting on your heels in Rock Pose. If you need to put a pillow between your butt and heels, that's totally fine. You can also do this in Easy Pose, sitting cross-legged, or in a chair.

Stretch the arms over head with elbows straight, until the arms hug the sides of the head. Interlace all the fingers except the index fingers. Cross right thumb over left for more masculine energy and left thumb over right for more feminine energy.

The spine stays still and straight through the whole meditation. Remain firmly seated on the heels (or in your modified posture) throughout the motions of the kriya.

We'll begin to chant "Sat Naam" with a constant rhythm—about eight times per ten seconds. As you pull the navel in and up toward the spine, chant "Sat" from the navel point (the energy center located two to three inches below the belly button). Feel it as a pressure from the third chakra, which is located at your navel point. With the sound "Naam," relax the belly.[53]

Eyes. Close your eyes.

Breath. The breath regulates itself, so just let it do what feels best.

Time. Continue for three minutes. You can work up to thirty-one minutes if you'd like!

To end. Inhale and gently squeeze the muscles from the buttocks all the way up along the spine. Hold the breath briefly as you concentrate on the area just above the top of the head. Exhale completely.

Inhale again, exhale totally, and hold the breath out as you contract the lower pelvis, lift the diaphragm, lock in the chin, and squeeze all the muscles from the buttocks up to the neck. Hold the breath out for five to twenty seconds, according to your comfort and capacity.

Inhale one last time and relax. Then, come down onto your back and relax, feeling the energetic changes in your body. Stay here for at least six minutes. It is recommended to relax after Sat Kriya for double the time you practice the kriya itself. Feel free now to pick up your citrine crystal and place it on your navel point while you meditate.

Seal your practice with Sat Naam. Bring your hands together in Prayer Pose in front of your heart. Inhale deeply and either chant or say out loud "Sat Naam," which means "truth is my essence."

Affirmation

Choose an affirmation from the list below that reflects how you want to feel about your masculine energy, or create one of your own. What would bring your masculine and feminine energies into balance and make you feel power- ful? Repeat this affirmation three to five times before you get up off of your mat and head to the kitchen.

I am at peace in my mind and body.

I am connected to and guided by the divine energy within me.

I am creating space to receive and hold more energy.

My power is in knowing when to take action.

My willpower is as strong as the sun.

Nourishment

Divine masculine energy is connected to the sun, the brightest light in our universe. Certain foods are also connected to the sun, like the oranges in this post-ritual smoothie. This is one of our absolute favorite recipes because it's detoxifying, reduces inflammation, and helps heal the liver and stomach. We've added the Ayuverdic herb shatavari, which promotes vitality, strength, a healthy libido, fertility in women, and sperm production in men.

Sun God Shatavari Smoothie

Prep time: 5 minutes
Makes 1–2 large servings

1 cup pineapple

2 navel oranges, quartered and peeled

1-inch piece fresh ginger, peeled

½-inch piece turmeric, peeled (or 1 teaspoon powdered turmeric)

¼ tsp shatavari powder

Pinch of black pepper and sea salt

1 cup almond milk

2 teaspoons almond or sesame oil

Substitution ideas: instead of pineapple, try mango or peach.

>> In a blender, mix all of the ingredients and blend well, until smooth. Pour into glasses and serve.

> **GO UNLEASH YOUR INNER SUN GOD WARRIOR ON THE WORLD TODAY!** WE NEED MORE PEOPLE ON THE PLANET WITH HEALTHY AND STRONG DIVINE MASCULINE ENERGY GETTING THINGS DONE AND BEING AN EXAMPLE FOR HOW WE CAN BE COMPASSIONATE AND CALM BUT STRONG AND FOCUSED ALL IN ONE.
>
> *—Sat Naam and XO, B+T*

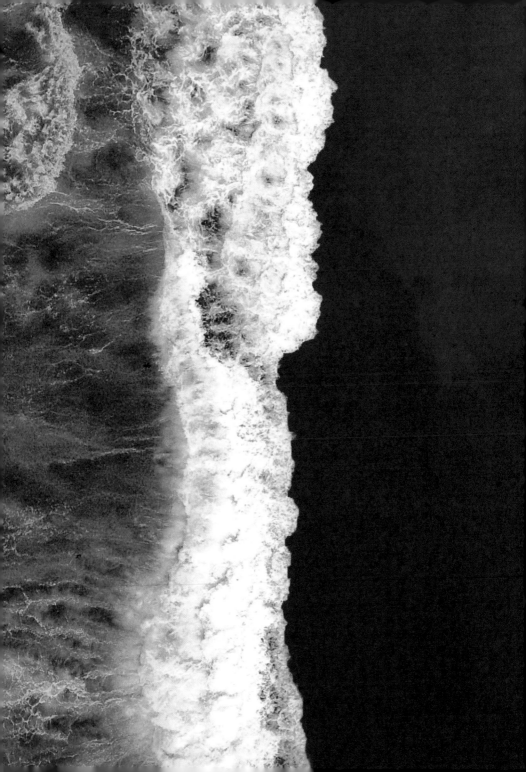

Elevate Yourself to Heal the Globe

We want to let you in on a secret: Your spiritual practice doesn't *just* benefit you. It kicks off a ripple effect that helps elevate everyone and everything around you...major bonus!

Since starting our morning rituals, many friends and family members have added spiritual practices into their own lives without any prodding from us—they were inspired to do so just from being around us and seeing the changes we've experienced. We would have never guessed Tara's mom would listen to mantras every day or that Britt's brother would have a consistent morning practice that helped him grow a wildly successful business. Britt's husband, who was eating carne asada every other night and had never been to a yoga class when she met him, became vegan and turned into an avid Kundalini meditator and conscious creator.

Even when we don't realize it, our positive energy affects people. It's so exciting when it starts happening all around you! If that isn't some serious motivation to get your bum out of bed and into your sacred ritual space each day, we don't know what is. Think about how different society would look if more people were being exactly who they are, sharing their gifts with the world, creating positive experiences, and feeling better, and in turn spreading joy to everyone around them. Sounds amazing, right?

Our wish is that this book changes your world—we want you to understand that you matter, you're deserving, and you're worthy of all that you want. We hope you take what resonates with you from these rituals and pass it on in your own way, because you will uplift others with your energy. That alone changes the world! Healing yourself gives others energetic permission to do the same. Every perception shift and every moment you move closer to the inner source of love, your soul creates a ripple effect that has no end.

We believe it's up to all of us to contribute positive energy to the world and take action to be a part of solutions to issues we are collectively facing. There's so much that can be accomplished when we come together as an elevated community to create change. Just look at organizations like Charity: Water, which has brought clean, safe drinking water to almost nine million people since it launched in 2006, or the Good Food Institute, which is working to promote humane, plant-based alternatives to animal products. Our friend, LaRayia Gaston, started Lunch On Me, a nonprofit that feeds healthy, organic meals to over ten thousand homeless people a month on LA's Skid Row and provides them with wellness services like yoga for mental health. These all started as ideas in the mind of just one person, and they've snowballed to make a massive impact.

We hope you'll realize that having a sacred morning ritual—raising your vibration with the rising of the sun—is the quickest way to raise the vibration of your life and make a positive impact on the world. With time, you will find a blissful place within where you are energized by life in new ways. Your morning ritual consistently allows you to release limitations, give and receive more love, create things that give back to society, and be a changemaker in the world. It's a gift you can show up for and unwrap every single day. It's absolutely the nucleus of our lives, and we can't wait to hear how you incorporate it into your lifestyle. (Reach out to us on Instagram or Facebook and let us know!)

It has been an honor to share these rituals with you! Our wish and prayer is that you will constantly come back and use them throughout your life, whenever you need them. Whether it's during a breakup, health issue, or point in your life when you are ready for expansion, you can always turn to these pages and commit to yourself again and again. We are always here for you and send you all our love and gratitude for being connected on this amazing journey of life with us.

—Sat Naam, B+T

Recipe Index >>>>>>>>>>>>>>>>>>>>>>>>>>>>>>>>>>>>>>>

Acknowledgments

Thank you, divine source energy, for the connection and flow of light that inspired this book and allowed it to come through us. Thank you to the moth in Big Sur that sacrificed life to spark this project. Huge thanks to our agent DJ Talbot, our amazing editors at New Harbinger, and to Erin, Siri Neel, and Miray. To our Kundalini teachers Colin Kim, Guru Singh, Tej, and Sat Devbir Singh—thank you for passing this technology on. We thank our families and dear friends for being cheerleaders along the way. Much gratitude to our ETG community for making this dream a reality—we do this for you.

"I dedicate this book to my amazing mother, Jennifer, whose soul drives my dedication to this work and who will forever be my motivation and guiding light. To my husband and soul mate, Justin, you make everything better in the world—thank you for love and support every step of the way. To Everest and Finnlyn, you are the brightest stars in my sky, and I hope you some day use this book and know that you can do anything." —*Britt*

"To my grandmother, Gail, thank you for sparking my interest in magic, energy, and the mystical at a young age. To my parents, Lorie and Dean, thank you for loving me without expectation. To my future family, my heart grows for you in every moment. To those reading this book: may it serve you at the deepest level of your soul and be a guiding light on this journey home." —*Tara*

Endnotes

Welcome to an Elevated Start, Every Day

1 J. F. Diaz-Morales, J. R. Ferrari, and J. R. Cohen, "Indecision and Avoidant Procrastination: The Role of Morningness-Eveningness and Time Perspective in Chronic Delay Lifestyles," *The Journal of General Psychology* 135 (2008): 228–240.

2 C. Randler, "Defend Your Research: The Early Bird Really Does Get the Worm," *Harvard Business Review* (July–August 2010), accessed February 1, 2020, https://hbr.org/2010/07/defend-your-research-the-early-bird-really-does-get-the-worm.

3 C. Wang, "These Men Think They've Discovered the Secret to Productivity," *CNBC* (May 5, 2015), https://www.cnbc.com/2016/05/04/these-guys-want-to-teach-you-how-to-meditate-help-you-be-more-productive.html.

Ritual 1: Natural Xanax

4 Anxiety and Depression Association of American, "Facts & Statistics," accessed October 30, 2019, https://adaa.org/about-adaa/press-room/facts-statistics.

5 N. Ramburn and S. B. S. Khalsa, "Yoga Research: Kundalini Yoga for Anxiety," accessed October 30, 2019, https://www.3ho.org/yoga-research-kundalini-yoga-anxiety.

6 S. Saiyudthong and C. A. Marsden, "Acute Effects of Bergamot Oil on Anxiety-Related Behavior and Corticosterone Level in Rats," *Phytotherapy Research* 25 (2011): 858–862.

7 D. Griswold, "Can Anxiety Be Caused by Dehydration?" CalmClinic (October 28, 2018), accessed October 30, 2019, https://www.calmclinic.com/anxiety/causes/water-dehydration.

8 "Meditation to Alleviate Your Stress," 3HO Foundation, https://www.3ho.org/ecommunity/2012/09/kundalini-yoga-meditation-to-alleviate-your-stress.

9 "Meditation to Tranquilize the Mind," 3HO Foundation, accessed March 23, 2020, https://www.3ho.org/3ho-lifestyle/health-and-healing/meditation-tranquilize-mind.

Ritual 2: Comparison Detox

10 This meditation was first taught on November 10, 2001; "Let the Self Take Care of Things," Sikh Dharma International, accessed March 23, 2020, https://www.sikhdharma.org/let-self-take-care-things.

Ritual 3: Let the Universe Take the Wheel

11 "Meditation for Self-Blessing and Guidance by Intuition," accessed October 30, 2019, https://www.libraryofteachings.com/kriya.xqy?q=crown%20sort:relevance&id=ad7d731b37ab446ba92cb1a397d43f22&name=Meditation-for-Self-Blessing-Guidance-by-Intuition.

12 A. William, "Healing Power of Melon" (May 10, 2017), accessed October 30, 2019, http://medicalmedium.com/blog/healing-melon.

Ritual 4: The Gold Rush

13 "Meditation for Prosperity II," The Yogi Bhajan Library of Teachings, accessed, March 30, 2020, https://www.libraryofteachings.com/kriya.xqy?q=prosperity%20meditation%20sort:r elevance&id=ba89a13b95a7431fbcba0d33e565d42a&name=Meditation-for-Prosperity-II.

Ritual 5: Shield Your Power

14 "Chii-a Kriya: Surround Yourself with Protection," 3HO Foundation, accessed October 30, 2019, https://www.3ho.org/kundalini-yoga/mantra/naad-yoga-how-mantra-works /chii-kriya-surround-yourself-protection.

Ritual 6: Shine Your Light

15 "Experiencing the Original You," 3HO Foundation, accessed October 30, 2019, https:// www.3ho.org/kundalini-yoga/pranayam/experiencing-original-you.

Ritual 7: Radiant Being

16 W. Hopler, "The Angel Diet: Foods that Raise Your Energy Vibration," (June 25, 2019), accessed October 30, 2019, https://www.learnreligions.com/ eat-foods-that-raise-energy-vibration-124708.

Pillar Three: Connecting to You

17 "The Precession of the Earth's Axis," accessed October 30, 2019, http://astrosun2.astro .cornell.edu/academics/courses/astro201/earth_precess.htm.

Ritual 8: Connect to the Divine

18 J. Arendt, "Melatonin and the Pineal Gland: Influence on Mammalian Seasonal and Circadian Physiology" *Reviews of Reproduction* 3 no. 1 (1998): 13–22; F. López-Muñoz, G. Rubio, J. D. Molina, and C. Alamo, "The Pineal Gland as a Physical Tool of the Soul Faculties: A Persistent Historical Connection," *Neurología (English Edition)* 27 (2012): 161–168.

19 D. X. Tan, B. Xu, X. Zhou, and R. J. Reiter, "Pineal Calcification, Melatonin Production, Aging, Associated Health Consequences, and Rejuvenation of the Pineal Gland," *Molecules* 23 (2018): pii: E301; M. P. Unde, R. U. Patil, and P. P. Dastoor, "The Untold Story of Fluoridation: Revisiting the Changing Perspectives," *Indian Journal of Occupational & Environmental Medicine* 22 (2018): 121–127; S. Seneff, N. Swanson, and C. Li, "Aluminum and Glyphosate Can Synergistically Induce Pineal Gland Pathology: Connection to Gut Dysbiosis and Neurological Disease," *Agricultural Sciences* 6 (2015): 42–70.

20 J. M. Bumb, C. Schilling, F. Enning, L. Haddad, F. Paul, F. Lederbogen, M. Deuschle, M. Schredl, and I. Nolte, "Pineal Gland Volume in Primary Insomnia and Healthy Controls: A Magnetic Resonance Imaging Study," *Journal of Sleep Research* 23 (2014): 276–282; W. Zhao, D. Zhu, Y. Zhang, C. Zhang, Y. Wang, Y. Yang, Y. Bai, J. Zhu, and Y. Yu, "Pineal Gland Abnormality in Major Depressive Disorder," *Psychiatry Research: Neuroimaging* 289

(2019): 13–17; N. Duggal, "5 Functions of the Pineal Gland," accessed October 30, 2019, https://www.healthline.com/health/pineal-gland-function.

21 E. Pennisi, "Cheetah Agility More Important Than Speed," *Science* (June 12, 2013), accessed October 30, 2019, https://www.sciencemag.org/news/2013/06/cheetah-agility-more-important-speed.

22 "Kundalini Yoga Varuyas Kriya," accessed October 30, 2019, http://www.pinklotus.org/-%20KY%20Kriya%20Varuyas%20Kriya.htm.

23 "The 4 Stroke Breath to Build Intuition," 3HO Foundation, accessed October 30, 2019, https://www.3ho.org/3ho-lifestyle/aquarian-age/4-stroke-breath-build-intuition.

Ritual 9: Activate Your Voice

24 "Meditation for the 5th Chakra," 3HO Foundation, accessed October 30, 2019, https://www.3ho.org/kundalini-yoga/chakras/meditation-fifth-chakra.

Ritual 10: Discover Your Destiny

25 Kundalini Research Institute, "Breath of Fire with Lion's Paws," https://www.kundalinirising.org/KRIResource/Meditations/BreathOfFire.pdf.

Ritual 11: Business Success

26 "Hast Kriya: Earth to Heavens," 3HO Foundation, accessed October 30, 2019, https://www.3ho.org/3ho-lifestyle/aquarian-age/hast-kriya-earth-heavens.

Ritual 12: Attract and Amplify Love

27 "Kriya for Creating Self-Love," 3HO Foundation, accessed October 30, 2019, https://www.3ho.org/3ho-lifestyle/authentic-relationships/yogi-bhajan-love/kundalini-yoga-creating-self-love.

Ritual 13: Magnet for Miracles

28 "Ego Eradicator," 3HO Foundation, accessed October 30, 2019, https://www.3ho.org/ego-eradicator.

29 Dr. Ramdesh, "Mantra for Positivity: Ek Ong Kar Sat Gur Prasad," accessed October 30, 2019, https://blog.spiritvoyage.com/mantra-for-positivity-ek-ong-kar-sat-gur-prasad.

30 "Meditation for Beaming and Creating the Future," 3HO Foundation, accessed October 30, 2019, https://www.3ho.org/3ho-lifestyle/aquarian-age/meditation-beaming-and-creating-future.

31 S. Layé, A. Nadjar, C. Joffre, and R. P. Bazinet, "Anti-Inflammatory Effects of Omega-3 Fatty Acids in the Brain: Physiological Mechanisms and Relevance to Pharmacology," *Pharmacological Reviews* 70 (2018): 12–38; "Do Omega-3s Protect Your Thinking Skills?" Harvard Health Publishing (November 6 2016), accessed October 30, 2019, https://www.health.harvard.edu/staying-healthy/do-omega-3s-protect-your-thinking-skills.

Pillar Five: Self-Love and Self-Care

32 E. Polack, "New Cigna Study Reveals Loneliness at Epidemic Levels in America," Cigna (May 1, 2018), accessed December 12, 2019, https://www.cigna.com/newsroom/news-releases/2018/new-cigna-study-reveals-loneliness-at-epidemic-levels-in-america.

Ritual 14: Addiction Rehab

33 J. Juergens, "Top 10 Most Common Addictions," accessed December 11, 2019, https://www.addictioncenter.com/addiction/10-most-common-addictions.

34 A. Bjarnadottir, "The 18 Most Addictive Foods (and the 17 Least Addictive)," Healthline (December 1, 2019), accessed December 14, 2019, https://www.healthline.com/nutrition/18-most-addictive-foods.

35 Guru Rattana, "Lesson 12: Breaking Addictions," accessed December 14, 2019, https://www.kundaliniyoga.org/lesson_12.

36 Yogi Bhajan, "Meditation for Healing Addictions," 3HO Foundation, accessed December 14, 2019, https://www.3ho.org/3ho-lifestyle/health-and-healing/meditation-healing-addictions-0.

37 C. N. Sawchuk, "Coping with Anxiety: Can Diet Make a Difference?" Mayo Clinic (May 24, 2017), accessed December 14, 2019, https://www.mayoclinic.org/diseases-conditions/generalized-anxiety-disorder/expert-answers/coping-with-anxiety/faq-20057987; Alina Petre, "18 Science-Based Ways to Reduce Hunger and Appetite," Healthline (June 3 2017), accessed December 14, 2019, https://www.healthline.com/nutrition/18-ways-reduce-hunger-appetite.

Ritual 15: Fountain of Youth

38 Administration for Community Living, "2017 Profile of Older Americans," accessed December 14, 2019, https://acl.gov/sites/default/files/Aging%20and%20Disability%20in%20America/2017OlderAmericansProfile.pdf.

39 Crystal Vaults, "Crystals for Youth," accessed December 16, 2019, https://www.crystalvaults.com/crystal-reference-guide/crystals-for-youth.

40 Yogi Bhajan, "The Whistling Breath," 3HO Foundation, accessed December 16, 2019, https://www.3ho.org/kundalini-yoga/pranayam/pranayam-techniques/whistling-breath.

41 Guru Rattana, "Kundalini Yoga Meditation to Become Young, Powerful, and Special," accessed December 16, 2019, https://www.yogatech.com/kysets/young.

Ritual 16: Healing Heartbreak

42 M. Laslocky, "This Is Your Brain on Heartbreak," *Greater Good Magazine* (February 15, 2013), accessed December 11, 2019, https://greatergood.berkeley.edu/article/item/this_is_your_brain_on_heartbreak.

43 Yogi Bhajan, 3HO Foundation, "Meditation to Heal a Broken Heart," accessed December 11, 2019, https://www.3ho.org/3ho-lifestyle/authentic-relationships/meditation-heal-broken-heart.

Ritual 17: Immune Upgrade

44 J. D. Sylvain, "Healing with Crystals: Improving the Body's Immune System," *The Mindful Word* (November 26, 2012), https://www.themindfulword.org/2012/healing-with-crystals-improving-the-bodys-immune-system.

45 Yogi Bhajan, *Praana, Praanee, Pranayam* (Espanola, NM: Kundalini Research Institute, 2006), 187.

Ritual 18: Energy Boost

46 Yogi Bhajan, *Praana, Praanee, Pranayam* (Espanola, NM: Kundalini Research Institute, 2006), 106.

47 Yogi Bhajan, "Eggbeater to Recharge Yourself," *Aquarian Times* (Spring 2004), accessed February 1, 2020, https://www.3ho.org/3ho-lifestyle/health-and-healing/eggbeater-recharge-yourself.

Ritual 19: Balanced Hormones

48 K. -B. Lee, Eun Cho, and Y. -S. Kang, "Changes in 5-Hydroxytryptamine and Cortisol Plasma Levels in Menopausal Women After Inhalation of Clary Sage Oil," *Phytotherapy Research* 28 (2014): 1599–1605.

49 Yogi Bhajan, *Praana, Praanee, Pranayam* (Espanola, NM: Kundalini Research Institute, 2006), 138–139.

50 F. Spritzler, "12 Proven Health Benefits of Ashwagandha," Healthline (November 3, 2019), https://www.healthline.com/nutrition/12-proven-ashwagandha-benefits#1.

Ritual 20: Feminine Support

51 Kundalini Women, "Call Upon the Maha Shakti," http://www.kundaliniwomen.org/med_Call_Upon_Maha_Shakti.html.

Ritual 21: Masculine Support

52 S. P. K. Khalsa, "Kundalini Yoga: Archer Pose," 3HO Foundation, accessed February 3, 2020, https://www.3ho.org/kundalini-yoga-archer-pose.

53 Yogi Bhajan, "Sat Kriya," 3HO Foundation, accessed February 3, 2020, https://www.3ho.org/sat-kriya.

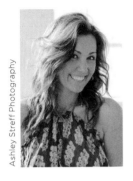

Ashley Streff Photography

Britt Deanda is a widely recognized Kundalini yoga and meditation instructor, speaker, and spiritual leader. She is cofounder, with Tara Schulenberg, of Elevate The Globe; cohost of a top spiritual podcast, *The Elevator*; cocreator of RISE UP: A Course in High Vibrational Living, and 528 Abundance Academy; and creator of The Conscious Bump. She is a conscious Mama, and activist for love and change toward a more elevated planet. Find out more at www.elevatetheglobe.com.

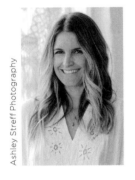

Ashley Streff Photography

Tara Schulenberg is a next-generation thought leader bringing spirituality to the modern world in a fun and easy-to-follow way. She is cofounder, with Britt Deanda, of Elevate The Globe, cocreator of the 528 Abundance Academy, cohost of *The Elevator* podcast, and Kundalini yoga instructor and astrologer bridging the gap between ancient wisdom and the modern world. Find out more at www.elevatetheglobe.com.

MORE BOOKS for the SPIRITUAL SEEKER

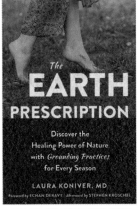

The EARTH PRESCRIPTION

Discover the
Healing Power of Nature
with *Grounding Practices*
for Every Season

LAURA KONIVER, MD

Foreword by ECHAN DERAVY | Afterword by STEPHEN KROSCHEL

ISBN: 978-1684034895 | US $17.95

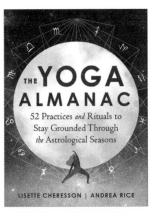

THE YOGA ALMANAC

52 Practices *and* Rituals to
Stay Grounded Through
the Astrological Seasons

LISETTE CHERESSON | ANDREA RICE

ISBN: 978-1684034352 | US $17.95

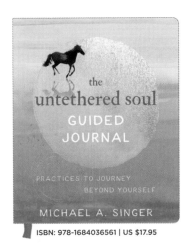

the untethered soul
GUIDED JOURNAL

PRACTICES TO JOURNEY
BEYOND YOURSELF

MICHAEL A. SINGER

ISBN: 978-1684036561 | US $17.95

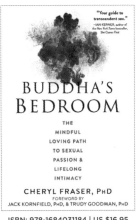

"Your guide to
transcendent sex."
—IAN KERNER, author of
the *New York Times* bestseller,
She Comes First

BUDDHA'S BEDROOM

THE
MINDFUL
LOVING PATH
TO SEXUAL
PASSION &
LIFELONG
INTIMACY

CHERYL FRASER, PhD

FOREWORD BY
JACK KORNFIELD, PhD, & TRUDY GOODMAN, PhD

ISBN: 978-1684031184 | US $16.95

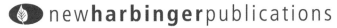

newharbingerpublications

REVEAL PRESS